General Chairside Assisting Exam Practice Questions

DANB®, CDA®, ICE®, COA® and RHS® are registered trademarks of the Dental Assisting National Board, Inc. (DANB). This product is not reviewed or endorsed by DANB.

Mometrix
TEST PREPARATION

DEAR FUTURE EXAM SUCCESS STORY

First of all, **THANK YOU** for purchasing Mometrix study materials!

Second, congratulations! You are one of the few determined test-takers who are committed to doing whatever it takes to excel on your exam. **You have come to the right place.** We developed these practice tests with one goal in mind: to deliver you the best possible approximation of the questions you will see on test day.

Standardized testing is one of the biggest obstacles on your road to success, which only increases the importance of doing well in the high-pressure, high-stakes environment of test day. Your results on this test could have a significant impact on your future, and these practice tests will give you the repetitions you need to build your familiarity and confidence with the test content and format to help you achieve your full potential on test day.

Your success is our success

We would love to hear from you! If you would like to share the story of your exam success or if you have any questions or comments in regard to our products, please contact us at **800-673-8175** or **support@mometrix.com**.

Thanks again for your business and we wish you continued success!

Sincerely,
The Mometrix Test Preparation Team

Written and edited by the Mometrix Exam Secrets Test Prep Team
Printed in the United States of America

TABLE OF CONTENTS

GC Practice Test #1

1. A small rubber stop is used in conjunction with a rotary hand file during an endodontic procedure for which of the following reasons?

a. To indicate the non-working length of the root.
b. To mark how long the master file should be.
c. To indicate what size file should be used.
d. To prevent perforation of the apex.

2. Which of the following demonstrates the correct way to take a patient's radial pulse prior to delivering dental treatment?

a. Ensure that the arm is at or below the level of the heart.
b. The patient should have the arm tucked in a flexed position as the pulse is being taken.
c. Have the patient stand up for maximum blood flow as the pulse is being measured.
d. The dental team member should palpate the pulse for a full two minutes to obtain an accurate reading.

3. When trimming a dental model, water is backing up and splashing over the guide table. What is causing this?

a. The study models have not soaked for an adequate amount of time prior to trimming.
b. The model trimmer is broken and should be taken out of service.
c. The reservoir beneath the guide table has become clogged with hardened gypsum.
d. The trimming wheel is in need of replacement.

4. Which of the following is a main function of saliva in the oral cavity?

a. Saliva helps to remove excess fluoride from the oral cavity, preventing fluorosis.
b. Saliva reduces the amount of acid produced by cariogenic foods.
c. Saliva speeds up the process of demineralization that occurs when foods are eaten.
d. Saliva helps to speed up the removal of food from the teeth.

5. What is the name given to the term that is used to describe how a dentist is generally responsible for the work and actions of all others in the practice?

a. Dental Practice Act.
b. Reciprocity.
c. Scope of practice.
d. Respondeat superior.

6. What should suture scissors be used for?

a. For cutting tissue.
b. For cutting suture material.
c. For cutting suture material and tissue.
d. For cutting suture material and gauze.

7. Which of the following is NOT part of the tray setup for dental sealants?

a. Etching agent.
b. Varnish.
c. Low-speed dental handpiece.
d. Pumice and water.

8. Which of the following instruments make up the "basic three" setup commonly used during an oral examination of a patient's mouth?

a. Endodontic explorer, mouth mirror, interproximal explorer.
b. Mouth mirror, explorer, cotton pliers.
c. Enamel hatchet, mouth mirror, locking cotton pliers.
d. Mouth mirror, U-15 scaler, cotton forceps.

9. What term is used in the dental office when scheduling patients to return for cleanings and routine oral care?

a. Recall appointments.
b. Automatic appointments.
c. Maintenance appointments.
d. Restorative appointments.

10. Which of the following is correct in regards to the HIPAA-required privacy notice?

a. It is a document explaining patient privacy practices and is given out to new patients only.
b. It has the main intention of providing patient health information to be used in public health research studies.
c. It is used to protect the patient's clinical records only.
d. It is a document that is used to set standards for the way patient information is handled and recorded in a dental practice.

11. The biting surface of the posterior teeth is called the:

a. occlusal surface.
b. incisal surface.
c. lingual surface.
d. mesial surface.

12. What is the name of the law that requires dental offices to have a written policy regarding patient privacy?

a. OSHA
b. Privacy Act of 1986
c. HIPAA
d. Dental Practice Act

13. When assisting during an endodontic procedure, which image is required to determine the length of the canal prior to the placement of the gutta percha material?

a. Initial endodontic radiograph.
b. Working length radiograph.
c. Final instrumentation image.
d. Root canal completion image.

14. Which of the following terms can be described as the process by which amalgam is formed by the mixing of the mercury and the alloy powders?

a. Trituration.
b. Postulation.
c. Activation.
d. Coupling.

15. Which age group develops bad dental habits that frequently need to be unlearned later in life?

a. Ages 5-8.
b. Ages 13-15.
c. Ages 16-19.
d. Ages 19-60.

16. After tooth removal, when is alveolitis usually found?

a. 2-4 days after removal of a tooth.
b. 1 day after removal of a tooth.
c. 2 weeks after removal of a tooth.
d. 12 hours after removal of a tooth.

17. Following the administration of fluoride, the dental assistant should instruct the patient to avoid rinsing, eating, or drinking anything for what length of time?

a. 10 minutes.
b. 25 minutes.
c. 30 minutes.
d. 45 minutes.

18. Bonding agents used in bonding amalgam to a prepared tooth preparation are:

a. of low viscosity.
b. of high viscosity.
c. applied after the amalgam has been placed.
d. applied only if there has been a pulpal exposure.

19. Which of the following choices is the best treatment in response to a patient who is feeling faint at the dental office?

a. Place him in the Trendelenburg position and administer oxygen.
b. Have the patient sit up and close his eyes and take slow deep breaths.
c. Administer nitroglycerin under the patient's tongue.
d. Have the patient use the epinephrine pen in his thigh.

20. What type of data will be found in a patient's clinical chart?

a. Patient address and phone number.
b. Copayment amount.
c. Insurance coverage.
d. Procedures being performed.

21. What is the name given to the heat that is produced by a gypsum product when it is in the process of setting up?

a. Exothermic heat.
b. Chemical heat.
c. Hygroscopic heat.
d. Indigenous heat.

22. What is the most common medical emergency that occurs in a dental office?

a. Syncope.
b. Angina.
c. Stroke.
d. Myocardial infarction.

23. When reviewing a chart, you notice that tooth #30 has a red "S" charted on the occlusal surface. This red "S" indicates that:

a. tooth #30 requires extraction.
b. tooth #30 requires an occlusal filling.
c. tooth #30 is sensitive.
d. tooth #30 is in need of a sealant.

24. Which of the following is used most frequently in a medical emergency?

a. Oxygen
b. Spirits of ammonia
c. EpiPen
d. Nitroglycerin

25. Which of the following statements is correct regarding the preparation and placement of non-eugenol periodontal surgical dressings?

a. The material comes in a single tube and a small amount should be expressed for each patient when needed.
b. This material can't be mixed and stored in advance.
c. Non-eugenol material has a long setting time when exposed to warm temperatures.
d. When placed, this type of dressing causes discomfort to the patient as it becomes rough when it sets.

26. What type of occlusion occurs when the jaws are closed and the occluding surfaces of the teeth are together in a way that produces maximum stable contact?

a. Functional occlusion.
b. Centric occlusion.
c. Malocclusion.
d. Distoclusion.

27. What position should hinged instruments always be placed in, during autoclaving?

a. The closed position.
b. The vertical position.
c. The open position.
d. The Trendelenburg position.

28. What measurements are reviewed in order to select the proper size dental dam clamp?

a. The facial width of the dental enamel junction.
b. The faciolingual width at the cementoenamel junction.
c. The faciolingual width at the cementoenamel junction and the faciolingual width of the dental enamel junction.
d. The faciolingual width at the cementoenamel junction and the mesiodistal width at the cementoenamel junction.

29. During which procedure will the dental assistant aid the dentist in the complete removal of the dental pulp tissue?

a. Indirect pulp cap.
b. Pulpotomy.
c. Alveoloplasty.
d. Pulpectomy.

30. When assisting during the placement of a stainless-steel crown, how can the dental assistant determine what size crown to place?

a. The correct size crown is determined by how the crown articulates with the teeth on the opposite arch.
b. The assistant must select the standard size for each tooth and use extra cement if the crown is too large.
c. It is the correct size when the prepared tooth has both mesial and distal contact with the surrounding teeth.
d. The dental assistant should try the crown on over the unprepared tooth prior to the start of the procedure in order to get the best sizing.

31. When the pre-measured amalgam capsule is over-triturated, the end result of the triturated mass appears:

a. crumbly and difficult to condense into the amalgam carrier.
b. crumbly and easily removed from the amalgam capsule.
c. mushy and difficult to remove from the amalgam capsule.
d. like the alloy and mercury are separate substances and have not been mixed.

32. A patient has finished his first visit for crown placement. The provisional coverage has been placed on the tooth in preparation for the crown placement. All of the following are appropriate instructions to the patient EXCEPT:

a. avoid sticky foods.
b. floss carefully and gently slide the floss between the temporary crown and the adjacent tooth.
c. be careful chewing in the area of the provisional coverage to prevent damage from occurring to the temporary crown.
d. if the temporary crown comes off, it is acceptable to wait until the next appointment to inform the dentist.

33. Which of the following choices best describes diabetes mellitus type 1?

a. The destruction of the thyroid gland leading to insufficient hormone production.
b. The condition that occurs with ingestion of too little sugar in the diet.
c. The body's attack on its own joints, leading to severe joint pain.
d. The body's inability to produce insulin.

34. In the positioning of the dental assistant for four-handed dentistry, which of the following is not recommended?

a. Eye level is positioned 4 to 6 inches above the dentist's eye level
b. Feet placed on the foot ring or base of the stool and the stool is positioned close to the dental chair
c. Legs are together, seating position is close to the back of the stool, feet planted firmly on the floor
d. Stool positioned close to the dental chair with legs parallel to the dental chair

35. What type of product is optimal for use in study models for the fabrication of a dental bridge?

a. Dental stone
b. Plaster of Paris
c. Alginate
d. Densite

36. Coronal polishing is contraindicated in which of the following situations?

a. A cooperative young patient.
b. A patient without sensitivity.
c. Poor health of the gingival tissues.
d. Orthodontic appliances present in the mouth.

37. Which of the following would be least likely to be found on the clinical examination form?

a. Temporomandibular joint (TMJ) evaluation
b. Dates of loss of primary teeth
c. Dates of tooth extractions
d. Information on crowns or bridge work

38. Which type of wax would be used to temporarily hold parts of a denture together during denture repair?

a. Utility wax.
b. Sticky wax.
c. Baseplate wax.
d. Casting wax.

39. Which of the following statements is correct regarding the use of a dental liner during an amalgam procedure?

a. It is placed after the amalgam restoration has been placed to seal off the amalgam material.
b. It is used to prevent the growth of secondary dentin that may disrupt the new restoration.
c. The brand name used during amalgam restorations is Copalite.
d. It serves as a thin barrier to protect the pulp from chemical irritation.

40. Which of the following may be contraindicated in a patient with severe hypertension?

a. Fluoride
b. Nitrous oxide
c. Levonordefrin
d. Lidocaine

41. What type of polishing agent should be used by the dental assistant when polishing a patient's mouth with a high number of aesthetic restorations?

a. Silex polishing paste.
b. Chalk polishing paste.
c. Coarse pumice polishing paste.
d. Micron-fine sapphire polishing paste.

42. Which of the following statements correctly describes the symptoms of a bronchospasm?

a. Pallor.
b. Polyphagia.
c. Short gasping inspirations and long wheezing expirations.
d. Disturbance of speech, vision, and swallowing.

43. Which of the following items must be included in the tray setup for a dental dam?

a. Dental dam punch, dam forceps, dental dam napkin, and dental floss.
b. Towel clamp, dental dam napkin, dental dam clamp, and U-15.
c. Dental adhesive, mouth mirror, scissors, and plastic instrument.
d. Dental dam clamp with ligature, dental dam napkin, dental hatchet, and dental spoon.

44. Demineralization occurs when which of the following three substances are lost from the enamel surface?

a. Phosphate, iron, & vitamin D.
b. Minerals, calcium, & phosphate.
c. Calcium, potassium, & vitamin D.
d. Minerals, magnesium, & vitamin B.

45. Where are paranasal sinuses located?

a. Behind the ears.
b. Behind the cheeks.
c. Within the skull.
d. Inside the maxillary palate.

46. Which of the following CANNOT be used as an endodontic root canal sealer?

a. Glass ionomer.
b. Zinc phosphate.
c. Zinc-oxide eugenol.
d. Calcium Hydroxide.

47. What is an easy way to visually identify a surgical bur from a general operative bur?

a. By the thickness of the bur.
b. By the length of the bur.
c. By the name of the bur.
d. By the manufacturer of the bur.

48. During an amalgam restoration, the axial surfaces of adjacent posterior teeth are removed. What dental instrument will be required to assist in restoring these axial surfaces?

a. A hemostat.
b. A matrix band.
c. An elevator.
d. A temporary acrylic material.

49. Which of the following describes an aura that is commonly experienced prior to a seizure?

a. The process of a patient becoming limp, clammy, and exhausted.
b. Temporary cessation of breathing.
c. Muscular rigidity and rotation of the head and eyes in one direction.
d. A strange sensation demonstrated by a certain taste, smell, sound, or sight.

50. When in centric occlusion, the distance between the labial surface of the mandibular anterior teeth and the lingual surface of the maxillary anterior teeth has an abnormal horizontal distance from that of class I centric occlusion. What is this condition known as?

a. Underjet.
b. Overjet.
c. Open bite.
d. Overbite.

51. Which of the following is NOT a function of a post-surgical periodontal dressing?

a. To provide protection of a recent surgical site.
b. To minimize the risk of infection.
c. To provide protection for teeth that may be mobile.
d. To minimize pain.

52. A patient who has had a heart transplant comes in for a dental procedure. He has a history of a penicillin allergy but needs to take prophylactic antibiotics prior to the procedure. Which antibiotic would most likely be prescribed?

a. Amoxicillin
b. Erythromycin
c. Ampicillin
d. Cephalexin

53. What is the difference between light-cured custom tray acrylic resin and self-cure custom tray acrylic resin?

a. Light cured custom tray acrylic resin sets as soon as it comes in contact with the monomer.
b. Self-cured custom tray acrylic resin sets when a light source is initiated.
c. Light cured custom tray acrylic sets via the initiation of a light source, while the self-cured custom tray acrylic resin sets when it comes in contact with the monomer.
d. The setting time is operator controlled.

54. When the dental assistant is planning the appointment sequencing of a partial denture creation, what should be scheduled to happen during the second appointment?

a. Complete a prophylaxis.
b. Select the shade and style of the teeth to be included in the partial denture.
c. Take preliminary impressions.
d. Expose radiographs and take any photographs that may be needed.

55. During instrument transfer, how should the dental assistant hold the instruments?

a. As close as possible to the working end.
b. In the middle of the instrument.
c. Three-fourths of the way up from the working end.
d. At the very tip of the non-working end.

56. The correct treatment in response to a patient who is hyperventilating is to:

a. administer oxygen.
b. have the patient cup her hands over her mouth and rebreathe her exhaled air.
c. lie the patient down and place her in the Trendelenburg position.
d. have the patient take rapid shallow breaths to get more fresh air into the lungs.

57. During the placement of dental sealants, which of the following protocols must be followed by the dental assistant to ensure that the sealant adheres properly to the tooth?

a. The dental assistant must ensure the tooth is completely dry prior to application of the material.
b. The tooth must be light cured both before and after the application of the material to allow for the sealant to reach its maximum setup.
c. Etchant should only be used on those teeth that have excessively deep marginal and central grooves.
d. All forms of moisture control should be avoided during the placement of a dental sealant to ensure the dental assistant has clear access to the tooth under treatment.

58. When evacuating during a restorative procedure, where should the evacuator tip be placed?

a. Approximately 2 teeth distal to the tooth being worked on.
b. Approximately 2 teeth mesial to the tooth being worked on.
c. Approximately one tooth distal to the tooth being worked on.
d. Approximately one tooth mesial to the tooth being worked on.

59. What type of procedure would include the following instruments: matrix set up, burs, saliva ejector, HVE, dental dam setup, and local anesthetic set up?

a. Extraction
b. Root canal
c. Class II amalgam restoration
d. Incision and drainage

60. Which gypsum product is also referred to as beta-hemihydrate?

a. Type III laboratory stone.
b. Plaster.
c. Orthodontic stone.
d. Type IV die stone.

61. Which of the following is NOT a test used to determine the vitality of a tooth prior to endodontic treatment?

a. Percussion testing.
b. Dry ice testing.
c. Laser testing.
d. Electronic pulp testing.

62. What is the proper ratio for mixing a noneugenol dressing?

a. 1 part base to 3 parts accelerator materials
b. 1 part accelerator to 3 parts base materials
c. 2 parts base to 1 part accelerator materials
d. Equal parts base and accelerator materials

63. What is the least effective strategy a dental assistant can take to assist a hearing-impaired patient in understanding instructions?

a. Remove mask before speaking to allow patient to see lips
b. Try to reduce other noise in the area when trying to communicate with the patient
c. Use written illustrations and handouts for the patient to read
d. Speak very loudly so the patient can hear you better

64. When the dental assistant is performing a coronal polish, what is the maximum amount of time the rubber polishing cup should physically remain on each tooth?

a. 30 seconds.
b. 15 to 20 seconds.
c. 3 to 5 seconds.
d. 10 to 15 seconds.

65. Which of the following techniques should be followed by the dental assistant when performing a coronal polish?

a. Use large amounts of abrasive agents to polish the teeth.
b. Apply very light pressure when polishing the teeth.
c. Ensure a very high rotation speed of the polishing cup.
d. Confirm that there is always polishing paste in the polishing cup when polishing the teeth.

66. When the dental assistant is punching the holes for the dental dam, what will happen during placement if the dental assistant punches holes that are too small for the patient's teeth?

a. The dam is not going to fit tightly around the teeth.
b. Saliva is going to easily leak through the teeth during the procedure.
c. The dam is not going to slip easily over the teeth and this will lead to tearing of the dental dam.
d. Excess material is going to bunch together between the teeth after placement.

67. If a dental patient has a seizure during treatment, the most important task is for the dentist to:

a. stop dental treatment and remove any disposable materials if possible.
b. secure the patient.
c. begin CPR.
d. begin the administration of oxygen.

68. When assisting the dentist, what instruments should the dental assistant transfer to the dentist during the removal of calculus from supragingival surfaces?

a. Scalers.
b. Curettes.
c. Hatchets.
d. Explorers.

69. When an unconscious but normally breathing patient is placed in the Trendelenburg position following a medical emergency, the body is positioned with:

a. the body in the supine position with the feet elevated slightly.
b. the head of the patient elevated, with the hands at the patient's side.
c. the arms of the patient held over the head.
d. the head between the knees.

70. Which of the following polishing strokes should be avoided by the dental assistant during a coronal polish?

a. The dental assistant should move the cup back and forth over the teeth without the cup leaving the teeth.
b. The dental assistant should always use a slow setting, applying overlapping strokes to the teeth.
c. The assistant should always establish a fulcrum, keeping the polishing cup close to the tooth.
d. The stroke should move from the gingival portion of the tooth towards the incisal edge of the tooth.

71. When holding a gingival margin trimmer upright, the cutting-edge forms a line that is parallel to the handle. This indicates that the margin trimmer is used on what aspect of the teeth?

a. Mesial.
b. Distal.
c. Buccal.
d. Lingual.

72. What is the chemical name of the abrasive that is used when operating an air abrasion unit?

a. Aluminum dioxide.
b. Aluminum monoxide.
c. Aluminum oxide.
d. Aluminum peroxide.

73. Mucogingival surgery involves all of the following, EXCEPT:

a. a vitrectomy.
b. covering exposed roots.
c. reducing muscle attachments.
d. reducing frenum attachments.

74. Which of the following is TRUE about the administration of nitrous oxide and oxygen (N_2O/O_2)?

a. The patient should be encourage to mouth breathe in order to maximize the effectiveness of N_2O/O_2
b. Once the dosage is determined for N_2O/O_2, the same dosage can be used at subsequent dental visits
c. The N_2O/O_2 procedure should end with the administration of 100% pure oxygen for at least an hour
d. Administration of N_2O/O_2 should begin with 100% pure oxygen

75. What method for ordering supplies would be used to obtain the best discount on dental supplies while having to stock only a part of the order at any one time?

a. Automatic shipments
b. Quantity purchase rate
c. Reorder quantity
d. Reorder point

76. During a routine surgical procedure, what is the correct order that the following instruments should be used?

a. Periosteal elevator, elevator, forceps, rongeur, bone file.
b. Elevator, forceps, bone file, rongeur.
c. Periosteal elevator, rongeur, forceps, bone file.
d. Bone file, forceps, rongeur.

77. Which of the following statements is TRUE about lubricant for the dental hand pieces?

a. It is universal in the use of all hand pieces.
b. It is only available for slow speed hand pieces.
c. It is universal for use only in high-speed hand pieces.
d. It should not be a universal product, and should only be used for the specific dental hand piece it was manufactured for.

78. During an amalgam restorative appointment, why might varnish be used?

a. To seal the enamel spindles.
b. To seal the cavosurface margins.
c. To seal the dentinal tubules.
d. To permanently cement a cast post.

79. What is the most likely reason that sealants fail?

a. The depth of the preparation.
b. The use of the wrong anesthetic.
c. Improper moisture control.
d. The amount of decay present.

80. When is a gingivectomy indicated?

a. To remove healthy tissue.
b. To remove periodontal pockets.
c. To clean the periodontal pockets.
d. To clean the interproximal surfaces.

81. Following an extraction, what instructions should the dental assistant give the patient in regards to brushing and flossing the teeth?

a. Use an extra-soft bristled toothbrush and brush the surgical site very lightly to remove food debris and bacteria from the area.
b. Instruct the patient to place a 2x2 piece of gauze over the area and then proceed to brush as normal and remove the gauze when finished to prevent infection.
c. Brush and floss the other areas of the mouth as usual, but avoid the extraction site.
d. The patient should brush and floss all areas of the mouth as he normally does to ensure that the bacterial content in the mouth is kept at a minimum to prevent infection.

82. Which of the following terms can be defined as profuse sweating?

a. Incontinence.
b. Diaphoresis.
c. Hyperglycemia.
d. Polydipsia.

83. When applying a topical anesthetic ointment in preparation for the dentist to give an injection, what is the longest length of time the topical ointment will provide optimal effectiveness?

a. 1 minute
b. 2 minutes
c. 5 minutes
d. 7 minutes

84. Which of the following is not an indication for a patient to receive a dental implant?

a. The improvement of the patient's appearance
b. The improvement of the patient's psychological health
c. To replace one of more missing teeth
d. To assist the patient with bruxism

85. When preparing and placing a provisional crown, which of the following should be avoided by the dental assistant?

a. Take a pre-operative impression and use this impression as a matrix to form the provisional crown.
b. Fill the impression matrix with the provisional material and place the impression back into the patient's mouth after the tooth has been prepped.
c. Allow the impression and the provisional material to remain in the mouth for a minimum of seven minutes to allow the material to set properly.
d. Cement the provisional restoration onto the tooth using a zinc oxide.

86. If decay is noted on the interproximal surfaces and the incisal edge of an anterior tooth, the classification of this decay is referred to as ________ decay.

a. class I
b. class II
c. class IV
d. class V

87. When assembling the anesthetic syringe prior to an injection, which of the following should be avoided by the dental assistant?

a. Hit the piston portion of the syringe with the palm of the hand to ensure engagement.
b. Organize and assemble the syringe and supplies outside of the patient's view.
c. Hold the syringe with one hand and load the syringe cartridge with the other hand.
d. Use finger pressure to engage the harpoon into the rubber stopper.

88. Which of the following is a NON-expendable item in the dental office?

a. A disposable item.
b. A light-curing unit.
c. A surgical blade.
d. A 27-gauge anesthetic needle.

89. What is the effect of chronic overexposure to fluoride?

a. Nausea
b. Diarrhea
c. Stomatitis
d. Fluorosis

90. When mixing zinc phosphate as permanent cement, where should the dental assistant mix the powder and liquid?

a. On a paper mixing pad to increase the mixing set time.
b. On a wax coated mixing pad to decrease the mixing set time.
c. On a warmed glass slab to increase the rate of the exothermic reaction and extend the mixing time.
d. On a chilled glass slab to decrease the rate of the exothermic reaction and extend the mixing time.

91. Which of the following conditions is characterized by a brain disorder that causes irregular output leading to convulsions?

a. Rheumatic fever.
b. Stroke.
c. Epilepsy.
d. Diabetes mellitus.

92. Which of the following statements is false concerning light-cured sealant application?

a. Poor sealant retention on the tooth surface may be due to contamination of the sealant with saliva during application.
b. Dental dams or cotton rolls will help to maintain a dry field when applying sealants.
c. Shining the curing light for 30 seconds will be the appropriate length of time to cure all surfaces that have been sealed.
d. Use floss to make sure there is no sealant in contact with the interproximal area of the teeth.

93. A patient who takes an anticoagulant medication every day may need to have their normal regimen altered because of which dental procedure?

a. A routine examination.
b. An invasive surgical procedure.
c. A single surface occlusal restoration.
d. Taking bitewing x-rays.

94. What type of instrument is used by the dentist to lower the height of the tooth during preparation for a crown?

a. Bevel instrument
b. Carver
c. High-speed handpiece
d. Ultrasonic handpiece

95. What name is given to the condition experienced by many pregnant patients who sit up too quickly in the dental chair after a procedure?

a. Hyperventilation.
b. Postural hypotension.
c. Cerebral hypertension.
d. Edema.

Answer Key and Explanations for Test #1

1. D: The rubber stop that is used in conjunction with the endodontic hand file prevents the file from being placed too far into the root canal of the tooth. If the file is placed too far into the canal, perforation of the apex of the root is possible.

2. A: A patient's radial pulse can be found on the inside of the wrist. It is best measured by having the patient sit down, have him put his arm at or below his heart, support the arm by a table or arm rest, and have him extend the arm straight out. It is common to measure the pulse for 30 seconds and then double that number to get the patient's pulse rate for one full minute.

3. C: When the reservoir beneath the guide table of the model trimmer becomes clogged with hardened set gypsum product, water that is normally circulating the trimming wheel also gathers in the reservoir beneath the guide table. This reservoir is equipped with an opening that allows for this excess water and gypsum slurry to exit the reservoir and empty into a trap beneath the sink. This tray ensures that the heavy particles of the gypsum are captured within the trap to prevent clogging of the water system.

4. D: When there is adequate saliva produced in the oral cavity, it helps to speed up the removal of food and debris from the teeth, therefore preventing demineralization from occurring and preventing decay. If there is too little saliva in the mouth, food will sit on the teeth for longer periods of time, and chances of decay increase.

5. D: In dentistry, the dentist is ultimately responsible for the work and actions of those team members employed in that dental office as long as those team members are practicing within their scope of practice. The term given to this description is respondeat superior.

6. B: Suture scissors should only be used for cutting suture materials. Using the suture scissors for anything other than suture material can dull the blades much more quickly than if they had only been used for their intended use.

7. B: Varnish material is not needed during the placement of dental sealants. This is a material that is used during the placement of amalgam restorations and serves to help protect the pulp. Sealants are only placed onto the enamel surface of the tooth, which should be cleaned prior to placement using pumice and water. The dental assistant must etch the tooth prior to placing the sealant material to prepare the tooth and allow for better uptake of the material.

8. B: When setting up for an oral examination, the dental assistant should have the "basic three" kit set out for the dentist. This kit includes the mouth mirror, explorer, and cotton pliers. The dentist will use these simple instruments to examine the teeth and may request others if needed.

9. A: Recall or recare appointments are those appointments for which the patient returns to the dental office every six months or some other specified amount of time to have his teeth cleaned and a possible exam by the dentist.

10. D: In 1996 the Health Insurance Portability and Accountability Act (HIPAA) was formed and is now used to set the standards for the way patient information is handled and recorded in a dental practice. It is set in place to protect all types of patient information and to allow for patient privacy regarding medical records.

11. A: The biting surface of the posterior teeth is called the occlusal surface. The incisal surface is the biting surface found on anterior teeth only. The lingual surface is the surface found closest to the tongue on all teeth, and the mesial surface is the surface that is found closest to the midline on all teeth.

12. C: The Health Insurance Portability and Accountability Act of 1996 (HIPAA) was enacted to help set national standards for the protection of health information. A dental office that transmits any health-related information electronically is required to comply with this law. This law also requires the development of a privacy policy for patients that must be reviewed with the patient and kept on file to acknowledge that the patient received and accepted the policy. Training for all personnel in the office is also required for safekeeping of patients' medical information. A policy regarding discipline of employees who breach patient privacy information is also required.

13. B: During the endodontic procedure there are a number of radiographs that are taken at different stages that aid the dentist in the correct placement of the final filling material. The working length radiograph is the picture that is taken to determine the length of the canal prior to the placement of the gutta percha material. After the canals have been filled, the root canal completion image is taken to ensure the material has reached the apex of the roots under treatment and that the procedure has been successful.

14. A: The process of trituration, also referred to as amalgamation, is when the alloy powders and the mercury found within an amalgam capsule are mixed together. This happens as a result of placing the amalgam capsule into an amalgamator which allows for the pestle found within the capsule to move back and forth at a high speed, mixing the other components in the capsule.

15. D: From the age of 19-60, many dental patients learn poor dental habits. Examples of such habits include using a toothbrush that has hard bristles, aggressive brushing, improper angulation of the toothbrush when brushing, and not using the toothbrush in a circular motion while brushing. Patients need education and encouragement to develop good dental habits throughout their lifespan.

16. A: Alveolitis usually occurs 2-4 days after the removal of a tooth. Symptoms will not occur immediately after the anesthetic has worn off, as the inflammation has not yet had time to sufficiently progress for the patient to be symptomatic. If the symptoms are present 2 weeks after the extraction of the tooth, the diagnosis would probably no longer be alveolitis but rather a persistent bone infection.

17. C: Following any type of fluoride treatment, the dental assistant should instruct the patient to avoid introducing anything into the mouth for at least 30 minutes to avoid disturbing the action of the fluoride on the teeth.

18. A: Bonding agents used in bonding amalgam to a prepared tooth preparation are of low viscosity. A low viscosity adhesive allows for the adhesive to flow into the cavosurface margins porosities present after preparing the tooth. A bonding material that has high viscosity is a material that is quite thick and does not flow freely. If a high viscosity bonding agent were to be used, the thickness of the material would create an open margin, because the material would not be able to flow freely into the porosities at the cavosurface margin.

19. A: When a patient is feeling faint, it is caused by insufficient oxygen to the brain, so in order to prevent fainting, have the patient lie back in the Trendelenburg position and administer oxygen. When the patient is lying on his back, this allows for the blood to flow to the patient's head, allowing the brain to get the oxygen it needs and helping prevent the patient from fainting.

20. D: A patient's clinical chart should include only the clinical information that relates to that patient. This includes any treatments that are being performed and any future treatment plans that have been proposed to the patient as well as the progress notes completed by the dental team members. Information including insurance coverage, personal contact information, and billing questions are all part of the patient's financial chart, not the clinical chart.

21. A: Exothermic heat is a type of heat that is produced when a gypsum product is in the process of setting up. This type of heat is generated due to the chemical reactions that are taking place between what is found in the gypsum products and the water.

22. A: Syncope is the most common emergency situation that occurs in the dental office. Patients are often apprehensive about their treatment while waiting in the dental reception area. Anxiety can cause changes in the patient's breathing pattern. Poor breathing habits produce poorly oxygenated blood from reaching the brain, which may lead to dizziness and eventually fainting.

23. D: A red "S" indicates that tooth #30 is in need of a sealant. A red "X" on the roots of the tooth of the dental chart diagram indicates the need for an extraction. A tooth needing a restoration on the occlusal surface would be charted as filling in the portion of the occlusal table in red on the dental chart diagram. A tooth that is sensitive to the patient will be noted in the clinical notes of the patient's chart.

24. A: Oxygen is used most often in a medical emergency. It is required for any patient who has is unresponsive but still breathing and is absolutely necessary for a patient who has stopped breathing. Portable oxygen tanks should be readily available in the dental office should the need arise for oxygen administration. Other drugs that should be on hand include spirits of ammonia for trying to arouse someone who has fainted, an *EpiPen*, *Chlor-Trimeton*, and *Benadryl* for an allergic reaction, and nitroglycerin for angina pain. Albuterol is required for bronchospasms or asthma attacks and *Valium* for seizures. A source of rapidly absorbed sugar should be available, such as orange juice or sugar, for a hypoglycemic reaction. Methoxamine (*Vasoxyl*) should be available for issues with blood pressure and atropine should be available for bradycardia.

25. B: Non-eugenol periodontal surgical dressing material comes in two tubes: a base and an accelerator. This material must be extruded at the time of each patient visit as it cannot be mixed and stored in advance of the patient visit. When exposed to warm temperatures such as the oral cavity, non-eugenol material has a fast setup time and is comfortable for the patient as it sets to a smooth surface.

26. B: A patient is said to be in centric occlusion when he is biting together and his teeth are in a position that allows for them to be stable, or produce maximum stable contact. This will differ from patient to patient as the teeth may be aligned differently. Malocclusion is a type of centric occlusion that occurs when the teeth do not line up well.

27. C: Hinged instruments must be placed in the open position while autoclaving. This allows for all areas of the hinged instrument to be properly sterilized. If the instrument is in the vertical position but not open, it is also possible that the instrument is not properly sterilized. Trendelenburg is a body position that a patient may be placed in during or after a medical emergency.

28. D: When selecting the proper size dental dam clamp, the faciolingual width at the cementoenamel junction and the mesiodistal width at the cementoenamel junction should be considered. Improper fit of the dental dam contributes to leaking around the neck of the teeth.

29. D: During a pulpectomy, commonly referred to as a root canal, the dental assistant will aid the dentist in the complete removal of the pulp tissue from the roots of a tooth. The root canal spaces will then be filled in using a filling material such as gutta percha or silver points.

30. C: When selecting the correct size of a stainless-steel crown, the dental assistant must use the relationships of the adjacent teeth and the stainless-steel crown to determine the proper fit. The crown is the correct size when it fits snugly on the prepared tooth and has tight mesial and distal contacts.

31. C: When the amalgam capsule is over-triturated, the end result is a mix that is mushy and difficult to remove from the capsule. It is important to follow the manufacturer's instructions when activating an amalgam capsule.

32. D: Placement of a crown typically takes 2 visits. The first visit includes selection of the appropriate shade for the crown, preliminary impressions, preparation of the tooth including core buildup and retention pins, and final impressions. The first visit also includes placement of the temporary crown or provisional coverage. It is very important for the patient to be aware of how important the provisional coverage is for the crown procedure. If any damage occurs to the temporary crown, it can negatively affect the final crown placement. If the temporary crown is damaged or dislodged, the dentist should be contacted immediately for replacement. Other instructions that should be given are to avoid sticky foods and to carefully chew in the area of the provisional coverage. Instruction on proper flossing should be provided. Floss should be gently slid between the temporary crown and the adjacent teeth below the contact to prevent damage from occurring. The second visit will include the cementing and finishing of the crown.

33. D: Type 1 diabetes can be described as a condition that results because the body is unable to produce insulin. If this is left untreated, a patient can accumulate too much sugar in the blood which can lead to severe health consequences. A patient who is suffering from type 1 diabetes must regulate his blood sugar by administering insulin into his body in some form; commonly insulin injections are given by the patients themselves.

34. C: Proper positioning for the dental assistant is extremely important. A specialized stool is used to help provide comfort and promote easy mobility while protecting against unnecessary strain to the upper body. The dental assistant should be seated towards the back of the stool, close to the dental chair, and legs should be parallel with the dental chair. The feet should rest on the bottom of the stool such as the foot ring. The eye level of the dental assistant should be 4-6 inches above that of the dentist or other type of operator such as dental hygienist.

35. D: Gypsum is the material that is used to make dental models used for orthodontic treatment, custom tray development, prosthetic devices, and the production of custom mouth guards. There are 3 forms of gypsum used. Densite (also known as improved dental stone) is used for the fabrication of dental bridges, crowns, or indirect restoration. Dental stone is used for the production of dentures. Plaster of Paris or model plaster is used for making preliminary impressions for orthodontic treatment. Water is required for nuclei of crystallization to occur. This promotes the growth of crystals during the setting process to provide strength and hardness to the final mold product. The ratio of water to powder is extremely important and requires careful measurement. For model plaster, the ratio is 100 g of plaster to 45-50 mL of water. For dental stone, the ratio is 100 g of powder to 30-32 mL of water, and for Densite, the ratio is 100 g of powder to 19-24 mL of water.

36. C: Coronal polishing should not be performed on a patient who has poor gingival health. The underlying cause of the poor health of the tissues must be addressed first, before coronal polishing can be performed. This is because coronal polishing will not be beneficial if the foundation of the teeth is not in a healthy state.

37. B: The clinical examination form is one of the most important forms in the patient's dental record. It provides very detailed information on past dental treatment, including location and dates of fillings, extractions, and crown and bridge work and other types of dental prostheses. The form also details examination of the oral cavity, soft tissue, overall oral hygiene, and condition of gums. Assessment of temporomandibular joint disorder is recorded here as well. Present and future planned examination should be recorded on this form. Any patient education is also documented on the clinical examination form.

38. B: Sticky wax is used to temporarily hold something together. This type of wax could be used during denture repair or when the dentist is working with models and the articulation of these models. This type of wax is very brittle when it is cold, but when heated, it becomes very tacky and sticky and holds things together well.

39. D: Dental liners are commonly used due to their ability to protect the pulpal tissue from irritation caused by chemical and physical elements. The liner that is commonly used during amalgam restorations is calcium hydroxide, with a brand name of Dycal. This material is placed into the deepest area of a restoration, followed by the restorative material.

40. C: Levonordefrin (*Neo-Cobefrin*) and epinephrine are vasoconstrictors that should be avoided in certain situations. A vasoconstrictor is a type of drug that causes the smooth muscles to constrict or narrow. This may cause undue strain on the heart or other organs. Patients with a history of severe hypertension, unstable angina, recent heart attacks or bypass surgery, or uncontrolled congestive heart failure should not receive a vasoconstrictor. Instead, an anesthetic without a vasoconstrictor should be used such as lidocaine or prilocaine HCl. Nitrous oxide can also be used. Another helpful consideration for patients with heart disease is to minimize the length of the appointment if possible, to avoid additional stress. Vital signs should be monitored and some patients may require supplemental oxygen during a procedure.

41. D: When polishing aesthetic restorations, the dental assistant needs to use a polishing paste such as micron-fine sapphire polishing paste, which is a low-abrasive paste that will not damage the aesthetic restorations in the mouth. Any polishing agent that has a fairly abrasive or coarse grit will damage and abrade the restorations in the mouth.

42. C: When a patient is suffering from a bronchospasm, commonly referred to as an asthma attack, he will experience short gasping inspirations or inhalations and long wheezing expirations or exhalations due to the inability of his lungs to process the fresh oxygen he is taking into his body. In order to treat this condition, the patient will need to use a bronchodilator or an inhaler to get the proper medication to his lungs in order to stop the spasms that prevent the body from taking in the oxygen.

43. A: When setting up for a dental dam placement, the dental assistant must include the dental dam punch, the dental dam forceps, the dental dam napkin, and dental floss with other instruments. If these items are not included on the tray setup, the dental assistant will not be able to prepare and place the dental dam in an efficient manner and will have to spend time during the procedure to leave the patient and gather these instruments.

44. B: The process by which the enamel surface has lost minerals, calcium, and phosphate is known as demineralization. Demineralization weakens the surface of the teeth, leading to sensitivity and an increase in the risk of developing caries or cavities.

45. C: The paranasal sinuses are found inside the skull. There are four pairs of paranasal sinuses: behind the nose, between the eyes, above the eyes and behind the sphenoid bones. They are air-filled spaces that are lined with ciliated respiratory tissue.

46. B: Zinc phosphate is not used as an endodontic root canal sealer. It should be used to permanently cement crowns and bridges on non-vital tooth structures.

47. B: Surgical burs are longer in length as they are often needed to reach into the tooth socket to remove fused bone that traps the tooth or root(s) in the socket.

48. B: During an amalgam restoration, the axial surfaces of the adjacent posterior teeth are removed. Restoring the axial walls of the adjacent teeth will require the use of a matrix band to help shape and create the new axial walls. The band will be made out of restorative material.

49. D: Many patients who suffer from seizures experience an aura prior to having a seizure. This aura could be anything including a certain taste, smell, sound, or sight, and may not always happen before every seizure. During this stage, the patient does remain alert and does not experience any physical body movements. These movements occur during a seizure, if one were to follow the aura.

50. B: Overjet is when the distance between the labial surface of the mandibular anterior teeth and the lingual surface of the maxillary anterior teeth have an abnormal horizontal distance when in centric occlusion.

51. D: Post-surgical periodontal dressings do not reduce pain after the procedure. They do protect the surgical site from mechanical trauma (such as from adjacent teeth) and infection.

52. B: Certain patients will require short-term or prophylactic antibiotics when preparing for a dental procedure. These patients include those with artificial heart valves, history of endocarditis, heart transplant, and congenital heart disease. Forms of penicillin such as amoxicillin and ampicillin are commonly prescribed. Cephalosporins, such as cephalexin (*Keflex*), are antibiotics that are closely related to penicillin. Patients with an allergy to penicillin should not be prescribed antibiotics from either group. Antibiotics that could be substituted in this situation may be erythromycin or clindamycin. Some patients do not tolerate erythromycin and may show symptoms of nausea or abdominal distress. This should be monitored and an alternative drug should be prescribed by the dentist as needed.

53. D: The primary difference between light-cured custom tray acrylic resin and self-cured custom tray resin is that the operator controls the setting time of the light-cured tray. First the operator manipulates the acrylic resin to the desired shape. Once that shape has been achieved, a light source is introduced, which will begin the polymerization process. Only after applying the light source for the recommended amount of time, will the polymerization process cure the acrylic resin. Self-cured custom tray acrylic resin does not set via a light source, but rather when the appropriate amount of monomer is added to the acrylic resin. After a specified amount of time that the monomer and polymer are together, a polymerization action occurs, resulting in a rigid final product.

54. B: During the initial appointment for the development of a partial denture, the dental assistant should plan on scheduling and assisting with a prophylaxis, taking preliminary impressions, exposing radiographs, and taking any pictures that may assist the dentist in the development of the partial denture. When the patient returns for the second appointment, the dental assistant will assist in the selection of the shade and mold of the teeth that will be included in the partial denture and will also help the patient and the dentist to fill out the lab prescription.

55. C: When transferring dental instruments, the dental assistant does not want to place his hand in the middle of the instrument, nor at the tip of the working end or the non-working end. The dental assistant should grip the instrument about three-fourths of the way up from the working end to allow for maximum stability.

56. B: When a patient is hyperventilating, it is due to having too much oxygen in the body and not enough carbon dioxide, and if this is not corrected it could lead to unconsciousness. The correct action is to place the patient's hands over her mouth so she can rebreathe her exhaled air in order to get more carbon dioxide back into the body. Oxygen should never be administered to a patient who is hyperventilating, as this will only aggravate the situation.

57. A: Prior to the application of a dental sealant the dental assistant must ensure the tooth is completely dry. If the tooth has any form of moisture remaining on it, this will interfere with the adhesion of the dental sealant and increase the chance that the sealant will fall off prematurely and render the tooth unprotected.

58. C: When evacuating during a restorative procedure, the evacuator tip should be placed approximately one tooth distal to the tooth being worked on. Water from the hand piece will follow a distal path in the mouth. Being as close as possible, without disrupting the working or viewing area of the provider, ensures that both patient and provider are comfortable.

59. C: A Class II amalgam restoration includes restorative tray containing basic setup, composite placement instrument, condensers, burnishers, carvers, and articulating paper holder. It also includes the setups for local anesthesia, dental dam, and matrix. High-volume oral evacuator (HVE) and saliva ejector are also included. Dental liners, base sealers, and bonding agents, as well as prefilled amalgam capsules, would be on the tray. The dental assistant would provide assistance to the dentist in the administration of the local anesthetic. During the preparation of the tooth for the restoration, the dental assistant would use the HVE and air/water syringes as needed to keep the area clear for the dentist to work. The dental assistant would mix the amalgam using the amalgamator and assist in the transfer of amalgam to the dentist. Assistance would also be provided as the amalgam is shaped, condensed, carved, and adjusted.

60. B: Beta-hemihydrate is also known as plaster. Plaster is composed of gypsum particles that are larger and more irregular particles than those of stone. Stone, although also included in the category of gypsum, is composed of particles that are smaller and are uniform in particle shape.

61. C: In order to determine the vitality of a tooth prior to engaging in endodontic treatment, the dentist may apply cold elements to the tooth. A necrotic tooth will not respond to the cold. The dentist may use electronic pulp testing to apply a stimulus to the tooth. If the tooth is necrotic, the patient will not feel any sensations. The dentist may also choose to use percussion techniques by tapping on the tooth with the mouth mirror handle to determine if there is any sensation felt by the patient. The use of a laser is not indicated in the determination of the vitality of a tooth.

62. D: Noneugenol is the most commonly used dressing in periodontics. There are 2 parts to the dressing: the base material and the accelerator. Equal parts of each type of material should be mixed on a paper pad. Using a tongue depressor, both pastes should be mixed until they are evenly distributed and the color is consistent throughout the paste. The paste can be prevented from sticking to gloves by coating the gloves with saline. Once the noneugenol dressing is mixed, it should be used immediately. Exposure to warm temperatures will cause the material to set very quickly.

63. D: A patient with sensory deficits, such as hearing or sight, can be challenging but there are steps available to address issues. For the hearing-impaired patient, simply speaking loudly is not a viable option. The dental assistant may not be aware of the degree of hearing impairment and it may be intrusive to other patients. Better approaches would be to make sure the patient can see the mouth and lips when speaking and to speak clearly and enunciate each word. It is best to try to reduce the amount of additional noise in the room when trying to communicate, such as the suction machine or television or music. Simple, concise instructions should be provided, and illustrations or handouts should be used whenever possible. In some situations, a sign language interpreter may be needed.

64. C: When performing a coronal polish, the dental assistant should only allow the rubber polishing cup to remain on each tooth for a maximum of three to five seconds. The longer the polishing cup is on each tooth, the greater the abrasive effect and the higher the chance that thermal trauma may occur, producing patient discomfort.

65. D: When polishing a patient's teeth, the dental assistant must ensure that there is always a small amount of polishing agent inside of the polishing cup. If there is too much polishing paste it will spatter, and if too little polishing paste is used more heat will be generated as the cup rotates in contact with the teeth.

66. C: When the dental assistant is punching the holes for the rubber dam, it is important to be sure that the holes are not too small. If the holes are too small for the patient's teeth, this will cause the dam to be difficult to place over the teeth and may lead to excessive stretching and even tearing of the dental dam.

67. A: During a seizure, the dental team must immediately stop all treatment. Dental instruments must be immediately removed from the mouth. Disposable products such as cotton rolls, gauze squares, cotton pellets, etc., should also be removed if possible. Patients should not be secured in any fashion, as this can cause the patient greater harm. CPR is only to be provided to a patient that does not have a pulse, or is not breathing.

68. A: When assisting the dentist during the removal of supragingival calculus, the dental assistant will set up and transfer to the dentist a variety of different scalers. The type of scaler used depends on the area of the mouth that the dentist is working in, as they have a wide range of angles and shaped ends to adapt to the curvature of the dentitions.

69. A: A patient who is unconscious but breathing should be placed in the Trendelenburg position following a medical emergency. The patient should be lying in the supine position, with the feet slightly elevated above the level of the head. This position encourages blood flows back to the brain.

70. A: When performing a coronal polish, the dental assistant needs to avoid moving the prophy cup back and forth over a tooth since this movement will cause excess heat to be generated and may produce discomfort for the patient. The assistant needs to use a slow setting and intermittent strokes when polishing to avoid trauma to the teeth and the gingival tissue.

71. B: A gingival margin trimmer looks like a chisel, but the blade can be curved either distally or mesially. When holding a gingival margin trimmer upright, the cutting-edge forms a line that is parallel to the handle, indicating that the margin trimmer is used on the distal aspect of the teeth.

72. C: Air abrasion units use a high-powered stream of abrasive powders to wear away tooth enamel and decay when prepping a tooth for a filling. This procedure allows the dentist to use smaller fillings and is generally less uncomfortable for the patient. The most commonly used abrasive is aluminum oxide.

73. A: A vitrectomy is not an example of mucogingival surgery, as it is focused on problems related to the retina of the eye. The goal of mucogingival surgery is to restore the function of the gingiva and to preserve healthy tissue. It can also be used to treat disorders of the gums or periodontal tissue, such as gum hyperplasia or loss of gum tissue.

74. D: Nitrous oxide/oxygen (N_2O/O_2) analgesia is also known as inhalation sedation. It has been in use since 1844. This type of sedation is administered through a nosepiece and is fast acting. N_2O/O_2 provides a very relaxing and good experience for the patient but can become habit forming if abused. A tightly fitting face mask should be used for administration and the patient should be instructed not to talk or breathe through the mouth to prevent nitrous oxide (N_2O) from escaping. The process starts with the administration of pure oxygen to establish the patient's tidal volume. N_2O is then titrated to achieve appropriate results. The dosage of N_2O can vary from one visit to the next; therefore, the dose must be reestablished each time. The N_2O/O_2 analgesia process should conclude with the administration of pure oxygen for approximately 3-5 minutes. The patient should be evaluated for the presence of headache, lethargy, or dizziness. If any of these symptoms are present, the patient should continue to receive 100% oxygen until the symptoms normalize.

75. A: Automatic shipments are a way for dental supplies to be ordered in bulk at a discounted rate. Only a portion of the order is shipped at a time, eliminating the need to find storage for a large bulk order. Supplies arrive periodically. Billing is also spread out over time, such as quarterly or monthly. Quantity purchase rate is also purchasing in bulk; however, typically the entire order must be received at one time. Ample storage space must be available for this type of ordering. Reorder quantity is the maximum amount of product that can be ordered at any one time and reflects frequency of use, shelf life, type of storage required, and availability of storage. Reorder point is the minimum quantity of a certain product that should be on hand at any one time. If the inventory goes below this number, the stock must be replenished.

76. A: During a routine surgical procedure, the periosteal elevator is used to loosen up the gingival tissue around the tooth. This will sever many of the gingival attachments beneath the cervical line of the tooth. An elevator is used next to uproot the tooth from within the socket and to allow for any additional attachments to be removed prior to lateral luxation of the tooth. After the tooth is no longer tightly held within the socket, the forceps are used to stretch and finally sever the ligaments attaching the tooth to the tooth socket. The forceps will also eventually remove the tooth in its entirety. Rongeurs may be used on the alveolar bone, if the periosteum has cracked while luxating the tooth. Once removed, the bone file may be used to smooth and contour the roughened area of alveolar bone.

77. D: Lubricant for dental hand pieces is made by the manufacturer for their specific product, and should not be used universally. Each manufacturer has specific maintenance schedules to follow for their products.

78. C: Varnish, when used in a restorative procedure, is primarily used to seal the dentinal tubules. Sealing the dentinal tubules assists in reducing post-operative sensitivity often felt by the patient who has had a restoration placed that extended into the area of the dentin. Varnishes do not have the strength to be used as permanent cement in dentistry.

79. C: The most likely reason that sealants fail is due to moisture on the tooth while applying the sealant. Sealants usually do not require any preparation of the tooth's occlusal surface; however, etchant is applied to the occlusal surface to prepare the enamel for receiving the sealant/adhesive materials. Anesthetic is rarely used while applying a sealant, as there is no preparation with a hand piece.

80. C: A gingivectomy is the removal of excessive or infected gum tissue. The procedure can be performed to clean the periodontal pockets by removing unnecessary debris from them. The excessive gingiva tissue is also removed to prevent rebuild-up of debris or food particles in the periodontal pockets.

81. C: After an extraction, the patient will have an open wound in his mouth until the area has time to heal. During this time, the patient should avoid brushing and flossing in this area, even with an extra-fine toothbrush. If he did brush over the extraction site, there is a chance he could dislodge a clot that has formed and open up the extraction site for infection. Nothing should ever be placed over or in the extraction site unless directed by a dentist.

82. B: Diaphoresis can be defined as profuse or excessive sweating. Many conditions can lead to diaphoresis, including nervousness and stress about the upcoming procedure, medications taken by the patient, and physical illnesses experienced by the patient. A dental assistant should stop the procedure if she notices her patient is experiencing diaphoresis and discuss what may be causing this, to avoid a more severe medical emergency.

83. B: Topical anesthetics are used before the injection is given to numb the nerve endings in the area of the injection site. Multiple forms of topical anesthetics include ointments, spray, patches, and liquids. The topical patch is the fastest acting agent at approximately 10 seconds; the other agents will start to work in approximately 15-30 seconds. The topical ointment is applied using a cotton tip applicator. The area where the injection will be given should be gently dried using cotton gauze. The ointment should be applied just below the injection site. The applicator should remain in place for at least 15-30 seconds and until the dentist is ready to give the injection. The longest length of time that the numbing effect will be felt is usually around 1-2 minutes.

84. D: A patient who has a history of bruxism should not be considered as a candidate to receive a dental implant. Bruxism is one of the top factors in implant failure.

85. C: When creating a provisional crown, the dental assistant should take a preliminary impression prior to the restorative procedure commencing. After the tooth has been prepped, the dental assistant should fill the impression with the restorative material and place it back in the mouth over the prepped tooth, letting the material stay in this area for an average of two to three minutes, allowing the material to reach its initial set. The impression tray can then be removed, the provisional crown can be shaped and prepared, and then it should be placed in the mouth using provisional cement such as TempBond or zinc oxide.

86. C: Class IV signifies dental caries that include the interproximal areas of anterior teeth and the incisal edge. Class V caries include the cervical gingival buccal or lingual areas of a tooth. Class II caries include the proximal surfaces of posterior teeth only. Class I caries include areas of development in the following three areas: a) lingual and buccal pits of molars, b) lingual pits of the maxillary incisors, c) occlusal surfaces of posterior teeth.

87. A: When assembling the anesthetic syringe, the dental assistant should never use the palm of his hand to engage the syringe as this could lead to fracturing of the glass cartridge that is home to the anesthetic. Instead, the dental assistant should use his finger and apply light pressure to engage the harpoon into the rubber stopper portion of the cartridge.

88. B: An expendable item in the dental office is one in which will be used for an extended period of time, with proper care and maintenance. A disposable item will be used once and thrown away. Both the surgical blade and the anesthetic needle will need to be properly disposed of by placing in the sharps container.

89. D: Fluoride is a mineral that is often added to water supplies to help with dental health. It is also present in toothpaste and children receive fluoride treatments as part of routine dental exams. Fluoride is also present in many foods in small amounts. Fluoride is considered safe at low levels but chronic overexposure to fluoride can lead to fluorosis. This can be seen as mottling or an opaque area on the surfaces of the teeth. Severe fluorosis can lead to deep brown pits on the teeth that look like decay. Acute or short-term overexposure to fluoride can cause nausea, vomiting, diarrhea, and pain in the abdominal area. In severe cases of acute toxicity, convulsions, irregular heartbeat, and even coma can result.

90. D: Zinc phosphate cement sets via an exothermic reaction as the monomer and polymer come into contact with each other. Mixing the monomer and polymer on a chilled glass slab ensures that the exothermic reaction is delayed, allowing for a more consistent final mixture. Decreasing the exothermic reaction allows for a longer working time while mixing and an increase in the quality of the final mix.

91. C: Epilepsy is a disorder of the brain that is caused by irregular output leading to seizures and convulsions. This can vary in severity and can be diagnosed by an electroencephalogram, or EEG, and can be treated and sometimes controlled by various medications. Seizures may be triggered by things including flashing lights, video games, and high fevers.

92. C: The sealant application process is very detailed. The surface of the tooth is first cleaned using a rubber cup and pumice or by air polishing the surface. Next, the enamel is etched using 37% phosphoric acid to allow the pores within the enamel to open up and accept the sealant material. Next, drying of the surface is extremely important. The presence of any moisture will cause the sealant to fail. A dental dam or cotton rolls can be used to maintain a dry field around the area. Light-cured sealants require the use of a curing light to cure or set the sealant. The light is shone on the surface for 20 seconds. Each surface that has received sealant application must be cured separately. Dental floss should be used to make sure sealant has not entered into the interproximal spaces. After the sealant application, the patient's bite should be checked using articulating paper.

93. B: Patients currently taking an anticoagulant should speak with the treating dentist about their medication regimen and whether they should take their anticoagulants prior to an invasive surgical procedure. Depending on the procedure, bleeding could quickly become out of control if someone is taking medication that prevents the blood from clotting.

94. C: Placement of a crown typically takes 2 dental visits. The first visit involves selecting the proper shade for the crown, taking initial impressions, preparing the tooth, and taking final impressions. Rotary tools such as the low- or high-speed handpiece are used to lower the actual height of the tooth as well as to properly contour the tooth so the crown will fit over the tooth and remain the same size as the original tooth. The first visit also includes placement of a temporary crown to protect the area being worked on. The second visit will include the actual placement of the crown for proper fit and cementing into place.

95. B: When a patient is pregnant and is in the reclined position for a dental procedure for any amount of time, she should be brought back up to normal positioning at a slower pace to allow for the extra blood in her body to flow back to its resting position. If the patient is brought up too quickly, the imbalance in the blood flow may cause the patient to become light-headed and possibly to faint.

GC Practice Test #2

1. Which type of medication would be prescribed by a doctor to a patient who is suffering from high blood pressure?

a. Antihypertensive.
b. Anticonvulsant.
c. Antipyretic.
d. Antiglycemic.

2. What is the name given to the excisional surgical procedure in which the dental assistant aids the dentist in the surgical reshaping and contouring of the gingival tissue?

a. Osseous surgery.
b. Incisional surgery.
c. Gingivoplasty.
d. Gingivectomy.

3. During an endodontic procedure, which of the following instruments should the dental assistant set out for the dentist to use to detect the pulp canals?

a. Endodontic explorer.
b. Endodontic spreader.
c. Broach.
d. Reamer.

4. Why must an alginate impression be left in a patient's mouth for the entire time specified by the manufacturer?

a. The impression will revert back into the gel state if not left in the mouth for the correct time.
b. The impression will develop air bubbles if not allowed to reach its final setting stages.
c. The impression will fall apart if taken out prior to its final set.
d. The impression will not be at full strength until that time period has elapsed.

5. Which of the following instruments will be used to pack in the amalgam material after it is placed within a preparation?

a. Enamel hatchet.
b. Amalgam condenser.
c. Football burnisher.
d. Walls 3 carver.

6. What type of plan is necessary to assist with repairs for frequently used equipment in a dental office?

a. Manufacturer warranty
b. Service contract
c. Equipment records including serial number and model
d. Extended warranty

7. Which of the following statements would be the most effective in communicating with an apprehensive patient?

a. The next sound you hear will be the drill.
b. We are preparing the tooth for restoration.
c. You will likely feel a little pain initially but it will subside once the anesthetic kicks in.
d. I am applying a topical anesthetic before the dentist comes in to give you the shot.

8. How is inlay, or pattern wax, used?

a. To create a die.
b. To create an impression tray.
c. To pour up a recently taken alginate impression.
d. To pour up a final impression.

9. Which of the following is the instrument that is used during surgical procedures to grasp soft tissue, bones, and remove any fragments that may have broken free during the procedure?

a. Forceps.
b. Scalpel.
c. Needle holder.
d. Hemostat.

10. You observe creamy white lesions that look like cottage cheese on the tongue and cheeks of one of your patients. This patient likely has:

a. herpes zoster.
b. herpes simplex.
c. lichen planus.
d. oral candidiasis.

11. Why would a dental assistant use a disclosing tablet prior to reviewing proper personal oral hygiene instructions with a patient?

a. To determine which teeth have restorations on them.
b. To demonstrate areas of decay to the patient.
c. To disclose areas of the teeth that may have heavy calculus on them.
d. To help identify areas where there is soft, sticky plaque attached to the teeth.

12. Key symptoms of a patient experiencing a myocardial infarction are:

a. loss of speech, dizziness, or weakness on one side of the body.
b. thirst, nausea, and twitching.
c. nervousness, fainting, and rapid breathing.
d. ashen color and diaphoresis.

13. Which of the following statements is NOT a reason why the dental assistant will use the high-volume evacuator during a dental procedure?

a. To keep the mouth free from saliva, blood, water, and any debris produced during a dental procedure.
b. To keep the tongue and cheek retracted and to keep the field of operation clear.
c. To remove all water from the patient's mouth after a full-mouth rinse by having the patient close the lips around the high-volume evacuator.
d. To reduce the amount of aerosol released into the air by the high-speed handpiece.

14. When assisting with the delivery of a partial denture, which of the following is NOT something a dental assistant would be responsible for?

a. Adjusting the tension on the retainer
b. Disinfecting the prosthesis before it is placed in the patient's mouth
c. Placing articulating paper in the patient's mouth in order to check the occlusion
d. Polishing the prosthesis before delivering to patient for instruction on use

15. Which of the following statements is INCORRECT regarding the application of a fluoride varnish by the dental assistant?

a. Dental floss may be used to guide the varnish material interproximally.
b. A cotton-tip applicator, brush, or syringe-style applicator should be used to apply the varnish to the teeth.
c. The fluoride varnish material comes in single-dose applications for the prevention of cross-contamination during application.
d. The patient's teeth must be dry prior to the application of the varnish material.

16. According to the Universal Numbering System, where is tooth 21 located?

a. Upper right cuspid
b. Lower right lateral incisor
c. Upper left 2nd molar
d. Lower left 1st bicuspid

17. A patient has just had a new permanent crown placed on tooth #16. What post-treatment instructions should be given?

a. Brush and floss the new crown and surrounding teeth carefully each day.
b. Use a mouth rinse with fluoride to improve the setting strength of the dental cement used on the crown.
c. Avoid flossing in the area of the new crown for one week to allow the cement to settle and prevent the crown from coming off.
d. Advise the patient to not chew anything sticky for five days to prevent the crown from coming off in the mouth.

18. Antifungal medications are prescribed to patients to treat which of the following medical conditions?

a. Thrush.
b. Hypertension.
c. Hypotension.
d. To prevent ovulation.

19. What is the name of the right-handed operating zone from 4 o'clock to 7 o'clock?

a. Operator's zone
b. Transfer zone
c. Assistant's zone
d. Static zone

20. What is the proper description of an anterior cross-bite?

a. The maxillary molars are lingual to the opposing mandibular molars.
b. The maxillary canines are positioned lingual to the opposing maxillary molars, when in occlusion.
c. The mandibular incisors are positioned lingual to the opposing maxillary incisors, when in occlusion.
d. The maxillary incisors are positioned lingual to the opposing mandibular incisors.

21. The air abrasion handpiece is least likely to be used in which of the following procedures?

a. Gingival retraction
b. External stain removal
c. Sealants
d. Class II preparations

22. During a composite procedure, which of the following actions should be avoided?

a. Prepare the tooth with etchant prior to placement of the composite.
b. Apply the composite in thin layers and cure between applications of these layers.
c. Select a composite shade one shade darker than the actual teeth to allow for dehydration during the procedure.
d. Polish the composite material after it has been light cured to its maximum setting.

23. When looking in a patient's mouth, the dental assistant notices that the patient's maxillary lateral incisors are missing along with the first premolars. What is the name of this condition?

a. Dens in dente.
b. Fusion.
c. Macrodontia.
d. Anodontia.

24. Bonding amalgam into a prepared tooth preparation assists with all of the following EXCEPT:

a. retention of the restoration.
b. decreased sensitivity.
c. decreased marginal leakage.
d. increased open cavosurface margins.

25. During an amalgam restoration, on what portion of the tooth is the cavity liner placed?

a. In the retention grooves of the preparation.
b. On the outer enamel surface.
c. On the lateral walls of the cavity preparation.
d. On the deepest portion of the dentin.

26. All of the following are true about plaque formation except:

a. the bacteria responsible for plaque formation are mutans streptococci and lactobacilli.
b. proper brushing and flossing can remove plaque.
c. the action of saliva will remove any remaining plaque following flossing.
d. potatoes and pasta promote plaque formation.

27. Why do dentists use a pulse oximeter during treatment?

a. To measure the oxygen saturation of the patient's blood.
b. To indirectly measure the patient's anxiety during treatment.
c. To measure blood pressure.
d. To directly monitor the patient's glucose level.

28. During an alveoplasty, what is the purpose of the rongeur?

a. To remove the impacted tooth.
b. To remove the remaining tooth fragments.
c. To trim the alveolus.
d. To trim the trigeminal nerve.

29. Which of the following is considered the most abundant mineral component found in the enamel portion of a tooth?

a. Lamellae.
b. Enamel prisms.
c. Osteoblasts.
d. Hydroxyapatite.

30. When working with a right-handed dentist, which of the following is the correct positioning for the dental assistant?

a. 7 to 12 o'clock.
b. 4 to 7 o'clock.
c. 2 to 4 o'clock.
d. 12 to 2 o'clock.

31. The permanent molars are:

a. nonsuccedaneous.
b. succedaneous.
c. of the primary dentition.
d. closest to the midline.

32. When a stainless-steel crown is placed over a deciduous tooth, which statement is TRUE?

a. The stainless-steel crown will remain in the mouth until the permanent crown erupts.
b. The stainless-steel crown will remain in the mouth for no more than 2 weeks.
c. The stainless-steel crown will remain in the mouth as a permanent adult molar.
d. The stainless-steel crown will be removable by the patient.

33. Through which duct does the submandibular salivary gland empty saliva into the oral cavity?

a. Duct of Bartholin.
b. Wharton's duct.
c. Duct of Rivinus.
d. Sublingual ducts.

34. What is the name given to the permanent teeth that grow in and replace the primary teeth in their specific locations?

a. Succedaneous teeth.
b. Deciduous teeth.
c. Tooth buds.
d. Exfoliated teeth.

35. Periodontal probes are calibrated in which of the following units of measurement?

a. centimeters.
b. inches.
c. micrometers.
d. millimeters.

36. The mouth-piece of the *Isolite System* is:

a. disposable.
b. autoclavable.
c. secured by the vacuum hose.
d. secured in place by the maxillary tuberosity.

37. Which procedure describes an osseous surgery that involves reshaping the bone?

a. An osteotomy.
b. An osteoplasty.
c. Bone grafting.
d. Periodontal dressing.

38. What is the correct action that should be taken when an impression tray fits a patient's mouth but does not completely cover the tuberosity or the retromolar pad area?

a. Select the next size larger and fill in excess areas of the impression tray with beading wax.
b. Add utility wax to the posterior borders of the impression tray.
c. Place boxing wax on the palatal area of the impression tray.
d. Place an excess amount of alginate into the impression tray to allow for more material to flow to the posterior portion of the mouth.

39. When breaking down a dental operatory after the patient has been escorted to the reception area, what is the initial step in the maintenance of the high-speed hand piece?

a. Remove the hand piece from the unit and take to the sterilization area.
b. Disinfect the hand piece and place the appropriate barrier.
c. Connect the hand piece to the unit and make sure the bur is in place. With the unit water on, allow for the hand piece to run for 20-30 seconds.
d. Connect the hand piece to the unit and make sure the bur is in place. With the unit water off, allow for the hand piece to run for 20-30 seconds.

40. If an oral tissue lesion is larger than 1cm in all dimensions:

a. an excisional biopsy is performed.
b. an exfoliative biopsy is performed.
c. an incisional biopsy is performed.
d. an alveoplasty procedure is performed.

41. Which of the following statements best describes how the dental assistant should use a surgical suction tip during a procedure?

a. The dental assistant should use the surgical suction tip to focus on extracting excess water from the patient's oral cavity during a surgical procedure.
b. The surgical suction tip is best used by the dental assistant to retract the lip during a surgical procedure.
c. The surgical suction tip should be introduced into the patient's oral cavity only at the end of the procedure to prevent the suction from allowing the dentist to view the surgical site during the procedure.
d. The dental assistant should place the opening of the surgical suction tip directly at the site of the procedure to remove any blood, tissue, or debris that is produced at the surgical site.

42. When assisting in the placement of a suture, the needle holder:

a. clamps the suture needle at the needle point.
b. clamps the suture needle at the beginning of the thread.
c. clamps the suture needle at the middle one third of the thread.
d. clamps the suture needle at the very end of the thread.

43. Which type of polishing agent is the best choice for polishing porcelain?

a. Sapphire polishing paste
b. Aluminum oxide paste
c. Silex
d. Fluoride paste

44. When viewing a Tofflemire matrix retainer, which knob on the retainer is responsible for adjusting the size of the matrix band loop?

a. The inner knob.
b. The outer knob.
c. The guide channels.
d. The spindle of the retainer.

45. Which of the following statements would NOT be a recommendation given to parents to help reduce the risk of cavity formation in their 8-year-old child?

a. Drink juice or water instead of soda
b. Avoid sticky foods such as raisins, dried fruits, granola bars, caramel, Skittles, and jelly beans
c. Offer cheese as a snack or part of a meal
d. Chew gum sweetened with xylitol.

46. When placing topical anesthetic, which of the following protocols must be followed?

a. Place a large amount of topical anesthetic onto a cotton-tip applicator.
b. If more topical is needed after placement, use the same applicator to gather more from the ointment container.
c. Place the ointment directly on the injection site.
d. Allow the ointment to sit on site for a maximum of one minute and then wipe off the ointment prior to injection.

47. What should be done with burs that are removed from the ultrasonic sterilizer, but have debris remaining on their flutes?

a. The bur should be disposed of.
b. The burs should be dried and properly bagged for sterilization.
c. The burs should be dried and placed directly in the autoclave.
d. The burs should be re-cleaned with a wire brush to remove the debris, followed by an additional period of time in the ultrasonic.

48. The purpose of using 2x2 sterile gauze squares immediately following an extraction are all of the following EXCEPT:

a. To control bleeding.
b. To promote healing.
c. To promote clot formation.
d. To control pain.

49. Which of the following choices is NOT a function of the periodontal ligament?

a. To protect and support each tooth in the tooth socket.
b. To provide nutrients to the tooth and surrounding tissues.
c. To protect the tooth from excessive nerve stimuli.
d. To supply fibroblasts to the ligaments.

50. You notice that your patient has indicated that they are taking an antilipemic medication as prescribed by their physician. What medical condition is this medication indicated to treat?

a. Hypothyroidism.
b. Hypertension.
c. Hyperlipidemia.
d. Arthritis.

51. When is a gingivoplasty indicated?

a. To remove periodontal pockets.
b. To remove periodontal ligaments.
c. To re-contour the gingiva to remove deformities.
d. To re-contour the tuberosity.

52. A micro etcher is most closely related to which type of dental hand piece?

a. The electric hand piece.
b. The high-speed hand piece.
c. The air abrasion unit.
d. The low speed hand piece.

53. Which of the following statements is correct when considering the use and storage of any gypsum product?

a. Wash excess gypsum powder into a standard sink when finished with the product.
b. There is no need for disinfection as gypsum products have natural antibacterial properties.
c. Store gypsum products in airtight containers.
d. Place gypsum products in the powdered form in moist, dark environments.

54. Which of the following products should be avoided during a composite restoration?

a. Varnish.
b. Prime & Bond.
c. Etchant.
d. Vitrebond.

55. When assisting the dentist with bonding orthodontic brackets, what type of glass ionomer cement should the dental assistant use?

a. Type I.
b. Type II.
c. Type III.
d. Type IV.

56. What is the best course of action to follow if a patient is suffering from a cerebral vascular abnormality or stroke?

a. Administer epinephrine from the epinephrine pen in the medical emergency kit.
b. Have the patient stand up to allow for blood flow to be directed away from the head to relieve cranial pressure.
c. Place the patient in the supine position and administer oxygen.
d. Keep the patient calm and call the emergency response team.

57. All of the following statements regarding the instrument tray are TRUE, EXCEPT:

a. Hinged instruments are placed on the tray so that the beaks are placed toward the assistant.
b. Angled instruments are placed on the tray with the primary working end of the instrument placed away from the assistant.
c. Straight shanked instruments should have the primary end placed away from the assistant.
d. Hinged instruments are not always placed on the tray.

58. Which of the following is a characteristic of arterial bleeding?

a. The most common type of blood loss.
b. Slow, oozing blood.
c. Dark in color.
d. Can cause death within a short time period if not stopped.

59. What are the three incisal bumps found on newly erupted permanent maxillary central incisors referred to as?

a. Cusps.
b. Mamelons.
c. Marginal ridges.
d. Supplemental grooves.

60. What of the following is most abundant in the human body?

a. Sodium.
b. Calcium.
c. Water.
d. Sulfur.

61. Which of the following is not located within the oral cavity?

a. Hard palate
b. Frenum
c. Gingiva
d. Pterygoid process

62. Which of the following statements is INCORRECT regarding soft drink consumption?

a. Diet soda is better for the teeth because it does not produce an acidic environment in the oral cavity compared to regular soda.
b. The sugar in the sodas combines with the bacteria in the mouth causing acid to form.
c. Soft drink consumption has been directly linked to dental decay, diabetes, and obesity.
d. Sodas have no nutritional value, with all of their calories coming from the sugars found in them.

63. When using dry-angle isolation, which of the following practices should the dental assistant consider?

a. Prior to the removal of the dry angle, the dental assistant should wet the pad with the air-water syringe.
b. It is common practice for the dental assistant to place a dry angle in the mouth first and then a cotton roll on top of the dry angle for the most efficient moisture control.
c. Dry angles are commonly used when working on the anterior teeth, and are placed in the vestibule area in the front of the mouth.
d. Dry angles are only to be used in procedures that have a risk of the high-speed handpiece and dental bur coming into contact with the patient's tissue.

64. When assisting a provider during dental treatment, the assistant inadvertently pokes a hole in her glove. What would be the first thing that the assistant should do?

a. Indicate to the provider that she needs to step out of the exam room for a moment.
b. Continue working to prevent disruptions.
c. Remove the glove and continue assisting the provider.
d. Put on a second glove over the torn glove.

65. The crown and root of the tooth meet at the:

a. apical one third of the tooth.
b. cervical line of the tooth.
c. contact area of the tooth.
d. cusp of the tooth.

66. When assisting with root canal therapy, what is the first instrument the dentist will need to enter the coronal portion of the tooth?

a. Carbide round bur
b. Endodontic explorer
c. Reamer files
d. Dental broach

67. Which of the following items is the most cariogenic?

a. Watermelon.
b. Soda/pop.
c. Raisins.
d. Potatoes.

68. When treating a patient experiencing a syncopal episode, what should the dental assistant do first?

a. Lower the head to increase blood flow to the brain.
b. Keep the patient supine but raise the head to increase blood flow to the extremities.
c. Have the patient sit upright.
d. Have the patient stand and raise the arms above the head.

69. A patient, on her health history form, indicates that she is taking nitroglycerin, as needed. What is nitroglycerin prescribed for?

a. Coughing.
b. A bacterial infection.
c. A viral infection.
d. To treat chest pain.

70. When assisting with a scaling procedure for periodontal debridement, what instrument is used by the dentist to remove supragingival and subgingival calculus?

a. Prophy angle
b. Kirkland knife
c. Gracey curette
d. Periotome

71. How should the staff communicate with a patient who is blind?

a. Written materials.
b. Body language.
c. Direct discussion with the patient.
d. Demonstration of important concepts.

72. When completing an amalgam restoration, which instrument is used to compact the amalgam into the prepared tooth?

a. Carver.
b. Burnisher.
c. Carrier.
d. Condenser.

73. During a fluoride application, which of the following steps must be completed by the dental assistant to ensure the fluoride is effective?

a. The dental assistant must dry the teeth with the air-water syringe or gauze.
b. The dental assistant must complete a full mouth debridement prior to the application of fluoride.
c. The dental assistant must supply a desensitizing agent to all teeth prior to application of fluoride to protect them from the negative effects of the product.
d. The patient must be in the supine position to allow for maximum comfort during the application of the fluoride.

74. Which of the following is the largest hole size on the rubber dam keyhole punch?

a. 0.
b. 1.
c. 6.
d. 5.

75. Which of the following dental dam clamps should the dental assistant select if performing a procedure on a mandibular molar in the permanent dentition?

a. W00.
b. W8.
c. W7.
d. W9.

76. In periodontics, what is the hoe scaler used for?

a. To remove supra-gingival calculus.
b. To remove restorations.
c. To smooth the cavosurface margin.
d. To smooth the root surface.

77. How should the dental hand piece fiber optics be cleaned?

a. A swab moistened with hand piece lubricating oil.
b. A swab moistened with isopropyl alcohol.
c. With a wire brush using soap and water.
d. With a wire brush using isopropyl alcohol.

78. In a dental office, a patient's health information may be released without her direct permission in which of the following situations?

a. To a company who is looking for a target group of patients to complete research on.
b. To a family friend who has made a verbal request on the patient's behalf.
c. To a healthcare provider or specialist involved in providing care to that specific patient.
d. To an insurance company that is seeking to complete an insurance estimate form.

79. Which of the following is NOT true regarding the application of topical fluoride foam?

a. Patients should be instructed not to swallow the fluoride
b. Patients may eat or drink right away
c. The teeth should be dry before the fluoride foam is applied
d. A double arch tray may be used to apply fluoride to both arches at the same time

80. Why are periotomes used?

a. To remove excess flash during a restorative.
b. To sever the periodontal ligament.
c. To remove the pulp from the pulp canal.
d. To sever the contact point between two teeth.

81. What type of wax is used around the periphery of an impression to form the base or the wall for the gypsum product that will be used to pour up the impression?

a. Inlay wax.
b. Baseplate wax.
c. Boxing wax.
d. Casting wax.

82. What is the term used to describe the amount of money that must be paid toward the cost of dental treatment before insurance benefits will be activated?

a. Deductible
b. Copayment
c. Benefit eligibility
d. Customary fee

83. When placing a dental sealant, which of the following would cause the finished sealant to have holes in its surface?

a. Too much sealant material was applied to the tooth.
b. There was saliva contamination during sealant application.
c. Air bubbles formed in the sealant prior to setup.
d. The sealant bite was too high.

84. Which phrase best describes bone grafting?

a. Adding artificial bone to an area.
b. Removing bone from an area and discarding it.
c. Removing bone from an area and moving it to another area.
d. Removing bone from an area and allowing it to encourage growth of additional bony material.

85. "T-Bands" are used during which dental procedure?

a. A pulpectomy.
b. An adult restorative procedure.
c. A restorative procedure of the deciduous teeth.
d. A prophylactic procedure.

86. The following statement is TRUE regarding the preparation of calcium hydroxide as a liner:

a. A small amount of both the base and catalyst should be expressed onto a large mixing pad.
b. A small amount of only the base should be expressed onto a small mixing pad.
c. A small amount of dental tray adhesive should be expressed onto a small mixing pad.
d. A small amount of both the base and catalyst should be expressed onto a small mixing pad.

87. Which of the following choices is the correct way to handle patient schedules and records in the dental office?

a. Have the patient schedule posted in each operatory and in the hallways so all staff members are aware of their patients for the day.
b. Have patient charts laid out in the front office by name so patients can select their chart when they walk into the clinic.
c. Store patient records and charts in the reception area in open storage shelves to allow for easy access when needed.
d. Place copy and fax machines in areas where other patients can't see what is being copied or faxed.

88. Which of the following are supplies found in a dental office that are quickly used during patient care and are frequently replaced?

a. Short-order supplies.
b. Non-inventory supplies.
c. Disposable supplies.
d. Expendable supplies.

89. Which of the following types of instruments should the dental assistant include as part of the tray setup which has the purpose of scraping the interior portion of a socket following an extraction?

a. Rongeur.
b. Forceps.
c. Surgical curette.
d. Elevator.

90. When measuring a patient's blood pressure, it is important to perform which of the following steps?

a. Have the patient stand up and rest the arm on a secure platform.
b. Center the cuff above the elbow and inflate the cuff slowly.
c. Place the stethoscope over the radial artery and hold it in place securely with your hand.
d. Inflate the cuff halfway and then release to capture recording.

91. When the dentist is completing a class III restoration, which of the following restorative materials will be used?

a. Amalgam.
b. Composite.
c. PFM crown.
d. Porcelain crown.

92. A posterior tooth is viewed as being tipped toward the cheek. Which of the following is the best term to describe this malposition?

a. Buccoversion.
b. Linguoversion.
c. Transversion.
d. Infraversion.

93. Which of the following is NOT an instrument that is used during an amalgam restoration?

a. Football burnisher.
b. Condenser.
c. Walls 3 carver.
d. Plastic instrument.

94. Under what level of supervision are dental assistants allowed to perform tasks within their scope of practice without the dentist needing to be physically present at the office?

a. Immediate supervision.
b. Direct supervision.
c. General supervision.
d. Indirect supervision.

95. Which of the following types of decay is commonly found in the elderly population due to the recession of gum tissue and bone loss?

a. Root surface decay.
b. Incisal decay.
c. Mesial decay.
d. Lingual surface decay.

Answer Key and Explanations for Test #2

1. A: When a patient is suffering from high blood pressure, she is said to be suffering from hypertension, so a doctor will commonly administer an antihypertensive medication to help in lowering the blood pressure. This may be combined at times with an antidiuretic that will allow for the body to remove excess water and therefore aid in reducing blood pressure.

2. C: During a gingivoplasty procedure the dental assistant will aid the dentist in the reshaping and contouring of the patient's gingival tissues. This is a type of excisional surgery in that it removes any excess tissue from the patient's oral cavity. During this surgery, the tissue is recontoured and formed to the desire of the patient.

3. A: During an endodontic procedure, the dentist will use an endodontic explorer to locate the pulp canals of a tooth under treatment. The spreader will be used to force the gutta percha into the canals, and the broach and the reamer are used to remove the pulp from the tooth and to enlarge the pulp canal space.

4. D: When taking alginate impressions, the dental assistant must leave the impression in the mouth for the entire time specified by the manufacturer of the material. If this is not done, the alginate material will not be at its full strength. When the alginate is setting up, it may appear to look ready to remove, but it must continue to remain in the mouth until the correct time has elapsed.

5. B: After the crown preparation has been finalized and the tooth is ready, the dental assistant will transfer a loaded amalgam carrier to the dentist, followed by the amalgam condenser. This instrument will be used to pack in or condense the amalgam into the preparation to ensure that there is no extra space left behind. The condenser comes in various sizes and angles to allow the dentist to reach all sizes and areas of all types of teeth.

6. B: Equipment records are important for keeping track of the model, serial number, date of purchase, and any servicing the equipment received. A service contract is critical to the smooth functioning of the dental office. If any of the key pieces of equipment break down, a service contract would help to ensure a quick response for emergency repair needs. Some service contracts will also include preventive routine maintenance. Manufacturer warranties are also important and typically cover repair or replacement for a certain length of time. Warranty information should be included as part of the equipment records. Another way to repair equipment is a service call. These tend to be expensive because the fee is based on mileage, amount of time required to repair, and the expertise of the technician. Service calls are typically used as a last resort. The cause of the issue should be explored thoroughly before making a service call, such as checking to make sure power is intact, check the reset button, or check the fuse box.

7. B: Dental fear or phobia is very real and how a patient is approached can make a big difference in future treatment. Verbal communication is very important. It is important to communicate with the patient in a way that he or she will understand. It is also important to make appropriate word choices to minimize the patient's reaction. Certain words, such as pain, shot, drill, or filling, may evoke fear or intimidation. Words that may be substituted include discomfort, anesthetic, prepare tooth, or restoration. These may be more effective. Nonverbal communication is also important. The patient is able to observe body language, so it is important to show a positive, stress-free image to the patient. This can be accomplished by breathing slowly and deeply, using calm facial expressions, and having an overall positive attitude. Good listening skills are also essential.

8. A: Pattern wax is melted on the die, which will form the wax pattern that is used to create the porcelain restoration. Beading wax, which is flexible, can be used to extend the length of an impression tray when taking impressions. Gypsum products are usually used to pour up alginate impressions, and to create study cast models. A stronger type of gypsum material is used to pour up the final impression.

9. D: The hemostat is an instrument that is used during oral surgery procedures for a variety of reasons. Some of these include aiding in the removal of tooth fragments that may have been produced during the procedure and also holding tissue and bone if necessary, during the procedure.

10. D: Oral candidiasis is an infection in the mouth caused by a yeast-like fungus named *Candida albicans*. It is also known as oral thrush. Symptoms include creamy white lesions that look like cottage cheese on the tongue or inner cheeks but may also appear on the gums, roof of the mouth, and tonsils. The lesions may bleed when scraped. If the lesions spread to the esophagus, difficulty swallowing may result. Patients who have a weakened immune system, have diabetes, or are receiving antibiotic therapy are at risk for developing this condition. Oral candidiasis is treated with a topical antifungal medication, such as nystatin, taken in the form of a lozenge or a liquid that is swished around in the mouth then spit out.

11. D: Disclosing tablets are used to determine areas on a patient that have high amounts of plaque on them. The teeth will turn colors in these areas, commonly indicating locations that are missed during normal brushing and flossing routines. Although some restorations and tartar in the mouth may turn colors when a disclosing tablet is used, this is not the purpose of these aids. It is to identify areas with higher amounts of plaque on them so the brushing and flossing techniques can be addressed and modified if needed.

12. D: An ashen color and diaphoresis are the key symptoms that patients experience during the beginning stages of a myocardial infarction. The loss of speech, dizziness, and weakness on one side of the body are classic signs of a stroke. Nervousness, fainting, and quick breathing are classic signs of a patient who in hyperventilating. Thirst, nausea, and twitching are signs of a patient having high or low blood glucose levels.

13. C: The high-volume evacuator is a strong suction that is used during most restorative procedures to keep the mouth free from saliva, blood, water, and any other debris that may be produced as a result of the procedure. This suction is very strong and the dental assistant should instruct the patient not to close his lips around the suction tip of the high-volume evacuator due to the discomfort that may be caused by the suction tip taking in the patient's tissues and tongue.

14. A: The dental assistant will lead the patient into the dental chair. After the prosthesis is scrubbed and disinfected, the dentist will place it in the patient's mouth. The dentist examines the fit and use of the dentures. The dental assistant places articulating paper into the patient's mouth in order to check the occlusion or the contact between the upper and lower teeth. Pressure indicator paste is also used to check for pressure points on the tissue that touches the prosthesis. The dentist makes appropriate adjustments for the comfort of the patient, including adjustment of the tension. Finally, the partial denture is polished and then thoroughly cleaned and disinfected before being given to the patient. The patient is educated regarding proper use and care of the partial dentures.

15. D: During the application of a fluoride varnish, the dental assistant does not have to ensure that the teeth are dry, as the varnish material is effective in the presence of saliva and is not moisture sensitive. A cotton-tip applicator, brush, or syringe-style applicator is commonly used to place the material onto the teeth, with dental floss commonly used to ensure that the varnish reaches the interproximal areas. The varnish commonly comes in single-dose applications to prevent cross-contamination during application.

16. D: There are three systems for numbering teeth. The Universal Numbering System is most commonly used in the United States. The mouth is viewed from the perspective of looking into the patient's mouth so when referring to the right or left, this should correspond to the patient's right or left. The mouth is divided into the following 4 quadrants: upper left, upper right, lower right, and lower left. The teeth are numbered starting with the upper right 3rd molar and ending with the lower right 3rd molar. The 3rd molars are teeth numbers 1, 16, 17, and 32. The 2nd molars are 2, 15, 18, and 31. The 1st molars are 3, 14, 19, and 30. The 2nd bicuspids are 4, 13, 20, and 29. The 1st bicuspids are 5, 12, 21, and 28. The cuspids are 6, 11, 22, and 27. The lateral incisors are 7, 10, 23, and 26, and the central incisors are 8, 9, 24, and 25. Wisdom teeth are considered 1, 16, 17, and 32.

17. A: When a new permanent crown is placed, the dental assistant must advise the patient to clean this crown as he would his normal tooth. Since it is a permanent restoration, the patient does not have to worry about the crown coming off from eating sticky foods, nor does he have to avoid flossing in the area. Using a mouth rinse with fluoride may help to strengthen other teeth, but will have no direct effect on the new permanent crown.

18. A: Antifungal medications are often used to treat thrush. Thrush is a fungal infection that is commonly found within the oral cavity, digestive tract, and skin of normal patients who have functioning immune systems. Taking antibiotics, high levels of stress, or an overabundance of yeast can contribute to thrush.

19. B: Operating zones were developed as a way to provide an efficient working zone that is comfortable and safe for the dental assistant and the operator (usually a dentist but could also be a hygienist). The operating zone is based on a clock concept where the patient's head is positioned at 12 o'clock. The transfer zone for a right-handed person is 4 o'clock to 7 o'clock. This is the zone where the dental assistant and dentist give instruments or materials to one another above the patient's chest. The operator's zone for a right-handed person is between 7 o'clock and 12 o'clock. The assistant's zone is considered between 2 and 4 o'clock for a right-handed person. The static zone is between 10 and 12 o'clock and is located behind the patient. If the proper zones are observed by each individual, the chance of bumping into each other is minimized.

20. D: A cross bite indicates that a tooth is not correctly aligned with the opposing tooth; therefore, an anterior cross bite involves malposition of the anterior teeth. Maxillary molars positioned lingual to the opposing mandibular molars indicates a cross bite; however, these molars are posterior teeth.

21. A: The air abrasion unit has been in use since the 1940s. The air abrasion handpiece is used for cavities and stain removal. Aluminum oxide particles are delivered via a high-pressure delivery system. This procedure removes enamel, stains, and other types of dental material without damaging the tooth. Local anesthesia is not required and is a gentler way of delivering care to patients. The air abrasion handpiece is especially effective when used for placement of sealants, access for endodontic procedures, crown margins, preparation of tooth for crown placement, and preparation of tooth for Class I through VI restoration.

22. C: Prior to a composite restoration, the dental assistant should select a composite shade that matches the patient's teeth color as exactly as possible. If this is done after the patient has had his mouth open for a long period of time, the shade may be off due to the dehydration of the teeth, and the composite may end up not matching the other teeth in the dentition.

23. D: Anodontia is a condition that causes one or more teeth in the oral cavity to be missing. This lack of teeth may be due to genetics, disease, or disruptions of the endocrine system during tooth formation. Dens in dente is a condition where a tooth bud starts to form inside of another tooth. Fusion is a condition in which two normally separate tooth buds fuse together during development, and macrodontia is a condition where a patient has abnormally large teeth.

24. D: The cavosurface margin is not made greater by the use of a bonding adhesive. Bonding adhesive is, in fact, used to decrease the microscopic openings remaining at the cavosurface margin, where the amalgam material was not able to completely fill.

25. D: During an amalgam restoration, the cavity liner must be applied to the deepest portion of the dentin by using a Dycal applicator, which allows easy access to small areas within a tooth. The liner must not be placed on the enamel, in the retention grooves of the preparation, or in the walls of the cavity preparation, as the main goal of the liner is to protect the pulp chamber.

26. C: Plaque is a clear, sticky substance that sticks to teeth. Two types of bacteria are responsible for plaque formation: mutans streptococci and *Lactobacillus*. This type of bacteria can be transmitted from one person to another. Proper brushing and flossing can help to keep plaque under control but saliva alone is not strong enough to remove or control plaque formation. A diet that contains a high amount of fermentable carbohydrates will contribute to plaque formation. Foods such as potatoes, pasta, bread, and sugar are considered fermentable carbohydrates. This means that when this type of food is consumed, the bacteria begin to feed on this and produce a byproduct that is capable of penetrating the enamel, leading to caries.

27. A: A pulse oximeter is used during treatment to measure the oxygen saturation of the patient's blood. Adequate oxygen saturation ensures that the patient is receiving enough oxygen and is tolerating anesthetics appropriately.

28. C: The rongeur is a tool with a spoon-shaped tip that is designed for cutting or gouging bone. During an alveoplasty, a procedure where the bone surrounding an extracted tooth is smoothed away, the rongeur trims the alveolus, or bony tooth socket.

29. D: Hydroxyapatite is the most common mineral component found in the enamel structure of a tooth. This is the mineral component that can be lost when a tooth undergoes decalcification due to dietary factors and decay. Hydroxyapatite minerals can also form in a tooth that undergoes recalcification by fluoride treatments.

30. C: When working with a right-handed dentist, the dental assistant will be positioned in the 2 to 4 o'clock zone. This allows for an adequate transfer space and also for a static zone in which the dental assistant can place her carts or instrument trays while allowing adequate room for both herself and the dentist.

31. A: The permanent molars are nonsuccedaneous. The three permanent molars (in each quadrant) are not replaced by the primary teeth, as they are posterior to the most posterior primary tooth. All teeth anterior to the maxillary and mandibular permanent first molars are deciduous and are normally succedaneous.

32. A: A stainless steel crown, when placed over a deciduous tooth, remains in the mouth until the permanent tooth crown erupts. Stainless steel crowns placed over deciduous teeth are primarily placed to hold the position of the adjacent teeth, which is necessary for the adult dentition to erupt. Often times during a crown and bridge procedure, an aluminum crown will be placed over an adult tooth that has been prepared for a final restoration, as a temporary restoration. The dental staff, in preparation for seating the final restoration, will remove this temporary restoration. Any restorative crown placed in a patient's mouth should not be able to be removed by the patient.

33. B: The submandibular salivary glands empty saliva into the oral cavity through Wharton's duct. This duct ends in the area of the sublingual caruncles. The sublingual salivary glands empty saliva into the oral cavity by means of the Duct of Bartholin. The Duct of Rivinus is also associated with the sublingual salivary glands.

34. A: Succedaneous teeth are the permanent teeth that grow in and directly replace the lost primary teeth. In the primary dentition, there are no premolars or third molars so as those specific permanent teeth grow in, they are found in different locations compared to the primary teeth.

35. D: A periodontal probe is a tool used to assess the health of the periodontal tissue and can help the dentist measure the size of lesions or the width of attached gum tissue. They are marked in millimeter increments along the working edge of the tool.

36. A: The mouthpiece of the Isolite System is disposable and should not be used again on a different patient. This reduces the possibility of cross contamination between patients.

37. B: An osseous surgery that involves reshaping the bone is known as an osteoplasty. It can be used to recontour and correct deformities of the gums. Bone grafting involves removing bone from one area of the gum and transplanting it a different area. Grafts can also be taken from animals or other human donor.

38. B: When an impression tray fits into a patient's mouth and covers all areas except the posterior areas of the maxillary or mandibular arch, the dental assistant can use utility wax and place this along the borders of the impression tray. This will then allow for the impression to capture the required structures without having to use an oversized tray.

39. C: When breaking down a dental operatory, the initial step in the maintenance of the high-speed hand piece is to connect the hand piece to the unit with a bur in place. With the unit water on, allow for the hand piece to run for 20-30 seconds. This action ensures that the airlines and water lines within the hand piece are flushed to eliminate any build up within the lines. This should be done prior to pre-sterilization of the hand piece. All hand pieces used in the operatory need to be properly prepared for sterilization and then sterilized. Disinfection of only the hand piece is unacceptable.

40. C: An incisional biopsy refers to the removal of an oral tissue lesion that is larger than 1cm in all dimensions. The lesion is sent to a pathologist who will examine the tissue under the microscope to look for abnormal cells.

41. D: During a surgical procedure taking place in a patient's mouth, the dental assistant will commonly use a surgical suction tip. The main function of this surgical suction tip is to remove any excess blood, tissue, and/or debris from the patient's mouth. The dental assistant will place the working end of the suction near the surgical site to allow for proper suction and to ensure the dentist can view the site without it becoming saturated with blood during the procedure.

42. B: The suture needle must be clamped at the beginning of the suture thread and at the very end of the suture needle. This allows the suture needle to remain rigid enough to pass through gingival tissues. Clamping the suture needle at the needle-point or in the middle one third of the thread will obstruct a portion of the needle and prevent it from passing completely through the gingival tissue.

43. A: It is very important to take the time to select the appropriate polishing agent. Polishing material is made of abrasive materials and is available in different degrees of coarseness called grit. The higher the amount of grit, the more abrasive the agent is. All polishing agents remove some enamel but the end result is to select the agent that will cause the least amount of abrasion. Sapphire or diamond polishing paste is the appropriate selection to be used on porcelain surfaces. Aluminum oxide should be used on hybrid and resin composites. Silex is an abrasive agent and should only be selected for teeth with a moderate to heavy amount of staining. Zirconium silicate is an agent that is less abrasive to tooth enamel than other choices.

44. A: When viewing a Tofflemire matrix retainer, the knob on the retainer that is responsible for adjusting the size of the matrix band loop is the inner knob. The outer knob is responsible for tightening and loosening the spindle against the band in the vice. The guide channels assist in directing the band to be held to the right or left of the retainer.

45. A: Many food-related tips or suggestions can be offered to parents to help reduce the risk of cavity formation. Water is the best beverage to choose over juice or soda because these contain sugar. Milk also contains sugar but does provide other nutrients important to dental health. Sticky foods, such as raisins, dried fruits, or granola bars, or chewy candy, such as Skittles or jelly beans, are not good for teeth. If the child eats any of these foods, the teeth should be brushed right away. Foods that stay in a child's mouth for a prolonged period, such as lollipops or hard candies, should be avoided. Including cheese as part of a snack or meal is good for teeth as it helps to increase the amount of saliva produced, which helps to cleanse teeth. Crunchy fruits and vegetables are a good choice for children. The use of sugarless gum or gum sweetened with xylitol helps to reduce bacteria formation within the mouth and to produce saliva.

46. C: When placing topical anesthetic ointment, the dental assistant should place a small amount of ointment on the injection site. Once the cotton-tip applicator has been placed in the patient's mouth, it should not be introduced back into the container due to the risk of cross-contamination. The dental assistant should allow the applicator to sit at the site for 15 to 30 seconds and then remove the applicator prior to the injection.

47. D: If a fluted bur has remnants of debris on it after being placed in the ultrasonic and run through a cycle, the bur should be re-cleaned with a wire brush and run through an additional cycle in the ultrasonic sterilizer. If the debris is not removed, the bur should not be considered sterile.

48. D: Sterile 2x2 gauze is used following an extraction to promote clotting and control bleeding. After extraction, the priority is to reduce and control bleeding. Pain control is not a function of the sterile gauze.

49. C: The periodontal ligament has a wide range of functions which help the teeth and surrounding tissues, and one of those functions is to supply nerve sensations to the teeth. This allows the teeth to provide a patient with a sense of touch when chewing foods, and the nerves found in the periodontal ligament also help to transmit signals to notify when an occlusion may be off during normal functioning.

50. C: Antilipemic medications are used to treat patients with hyperlipidemia, also referred to as high cholesterol. Patients taking certain antilipemic are at a higher risk for developing dental abscesses. In addition, some drugs can cause altered taste, leading the patient to increase their intake of sweet/salty foods and eventually increasing their risk for developing dental caries.

51. C: Gingivoplasty is used to reshape the gingiva to correct abnormalities of or to recontour the profile of the gingiva. This can be done for either cosmetic or functional reasons. Gingivectomy, on the other hand, is the removal of excessive or infected gum tissue.

52. C: A micro etcher is most closely related to the air abrasion unit. Both types remove small amounts of surface materials by emitting a substance onto the surface using pressure.

53. C: When working with any gypsum product, it is important to place any unused portion into the trash and not to wash it down the drain as this powder may react with the water and harden to clog the drain. After gypsum products have been used, they may need to be disinfected with iodophor solutions to prevent cross-contamination. Gypsum is also sensitive to changes in temperature and humidity, and should be stored in airtight containers in cool, dry areas.

54. A: Due to their ability to interfere with the bonding and setting reactions of composite materials, dental varnishes should not be used during composite restorations. The dental assistant will utilize these materials during an amalgam restoration as these materials are compatible with each other.

55. A: Type I glass ionomer cement is commonly used to bond on orthodontic brackets as well as cement on metallic restorations. Type II glass ionomer cement is used to restore areas of the teeth near the cervical area, and type III glass ionomer cement commonly serves as a dental liner.

56. D: A stroke can be caused by a blood clot blocking off a vessel or a vessel bursting in the brain. Any time that a stroke is suspected in a patient, it is imperative to get the emergency response team to the scene as soon as possible because every minute counts in the patient's prognosis. The patient should be kept still and the airway should be kept open, if the patient is unconscious, until the emergency response team arrives.

57. C: The only statement that is incorrect is that straight-shanked instruments should have the primary end of the instrument facing away from the tray. This is a false statement, because the primary end of the straight-shanked instruments should be placed toward the assistant.

58. D: Arterial bleeding is a result of one of the main arteries of the body being severed or cut. If this type of bleeding is not stopped immediately, it can cause the patient to bleed out in a very short amount of time, causing death. This type of blood loss is typically characterized by bright red blood leaving the body in spurting or pulsating patterns due to the proximity of the arteries to the heart.

59. B: The three incisal bumps found on the newly erupted permanent maxillary central incisors are referred to as mamelons. The anterior permanent teeth do not have any cusps present. Incisal edges and cingulum are found on the anterior teeth. Marginal ridges can be found on both anterior and posterior teeth, but not on the incisal edge. Supplemental grooves are located on the occlusal surfaces of posterior teeth, lateral to the triangular ridge.

60. C: Water is the most abundant nutrient in the human body. Chronic dehydration (inadequate intake of water) can lead to many health problems, including electrolyte imbalance, poor gingival health and salivary insufficiency.

61. D: The pterygoid process is located in the skull but not within the oral cavity. The oral cavity is the area located within the mouth. The lips are the entrance to the oral cavity. Parts of the oral cavity include the vestibule and the labial, which includes the frenum. It also includes the gingival or gums. The oral cavity proper refers to the area within the oral cavity that can be found inside of the dental arches. It includes the hard and soft palates, the tongue, taste buds, and teeth. The uvula is located within the oral cavity and is part of the soft palate.

62. A: Diet soda, commonly known as sugar-free soda, does not contain sugar but does contain high amounts of acid. When this acid is introduced into the oral cavity it attacks the enamel surfaces of the teeth and any exposed roots, causing demineralization. When consumed, each acid attack on the teeth can last up to 20 minutes in length, leading to weakened teeth and enamel.

63. A: Due to the manner in which the dry angle adheres to the patient's tissue in the mouth, the dental assistant should always thoroughly wet the dry angle with the air-water syringe prior to removal to avoid patient discomfort. The dry angle does not need to be used with a cotton roll as the dry angle itself produces sufficient moisture protection. Dry angles are commonly used in the posterior areas of the mouth, blocking salivary gland ducts and preventing excess saliva from entering the patient's mouth.

64. A: Should an assistant notice that they have a perforation in their glove during treatment, they should professionally notify the provider that they need to be excused for a moment. The assistant should then remove their gloves and discard them, wash and dry their hands, and put on a clean pair of gloves.

65. B: The anatomical crown and root meet at the cervical line of the tooth. The anatomical crown is the portion of the crown that is covered in enamel. Where the enamel ends and the cementum begins is known as the cervical line. The apical one third of the tooth will be located in the area of the lower one third of the root tip. Where two teeth touch is known as the contact area, or contact point. The cusp of a tooth is a point of elevation found on the coronal portion of a tooth.

66. A: Root canal therapy involves removing the dental pulp and replacing it with dental material. The dentist will need the carbide round bur to enter into the coronal part of the tooth to start the process of removing the decay and inner structure of the tooth. The next instrument will be the endodontic explorer and other intracanal instruments. These instruments may include endodontic spoon excavator, spreaders, and pluggers, which are used in the obturation of the canal. A Glick no. 1 instrument is used to place the temporary restorations. There are a variety of files, both hand and rotary operated, that will also be used within the pulpal cavity, such as the K-type file, Hedstrom file, Reamer file, and broaches.

67. C: Foods that stick or adhere to the teeth pose the highest cariogenic risk to the teeth. When a patient consumes beverages such as soda or pop, these do create an acidic environment in the oral cavity, but it is short lived. When we consume sugary items including raisins, these not only expose our teeth to high amounts of sugar, but these types of foods stick to our teeth for longer periods of time, therefore allowing for more demineralization and higher rates of decay.

68. A: A patient who experiences an episode of syncope should be placed in a position that raises the feet above the level of the head to increase blood flow to the brain. When a person faints, the brain experiences a decrease in blood flow. This causes the patient to briefly experience light-headedness with the loss of consciousness.

69. D: Nitroglycerin is normally taken by a patient to relieve chest pain. This medication is used to dilate the blood vessels in the chest to decrease pressure. While the symptoms of a viral infection can be treated, the infection itself cannot be cured by medication. A bacterial infection is usually treated with an antibiotic.

70. C: Periodontics is the treatment of diseases pertaining to tissues within the mouth, such as the gums. A periodontal exam is much like a regular dental exam, which includes a medical and dental history, x-rays, and oral examination. There are specialized instruments used for periodontal procedures, such as scaling, root planing, and periodontal surgery. Periodontal probes measure the depth of periodontal pockets and periodontal explorers are used to find the location of calculus deposits on the supragingival or subgingival surfaces. Scaling is the removal of supragingival or subgingival calculus from teeth. Curettes are used to remove deposits on the subgingival and supragingival surfaces. Two types of curettes are the universal and the Gracey. Scalers are also used for this purpose and the main difference between curettes and scalers are the shape. Curettes are rounded and scalers have a pointed end. Root planing is the procedure that removes the remainder of the calculus and smoothes the surface to make cleaning of the area easier.

71. C: When communicating with a patient who is blind, the staff should discuss important topics directly with him. All of the other possible answers rely on the patient being able to see.

72. D: The amalgam condenser is the dental instrument that is used to place and compact the amalgam filling material into the prepared area of the tooth. The condenser comes in different sizes to allow for ease of use with different-sized preparations.

73. A: Prior to the application of a fluoride treatment, the dental assistant must ensure that the patient's teeth are dry by using the air-water syringe or by physically drying the teeth with some gauze. This will ensure that the fluoride is able to work at maximum strength and the patient will get the most out of the fluoride application.

74. D: The rubber dam keyhole punch has a variety of punch sizes that can be used when preparing the rubber dam holes. The largest hole is size #5 and this size is used to punch the holes for the molar teeth, with the smaller sizes used for the canines and the anterior teeth. If the incorrect size is used to punch the dental dam holes, this may lead to the dam being too large or too small and may lead to interference with saliva during the dental procedure.

75. C: The W7 clamp should be selected when the dental assistant is working on a mandibular molar tooth in the permanent dentition as the 7 and the W7 clamps are standard for this area. The W00 clamp is commonly used in the primary dentition, the W8 clamp is a standard permanent maxillary molar clamp, and the W9 is a clamp used on the anterior teeth.

76. D: In periodontics, the hoe scaler is used specifically for smoothing the root surfaces of teeth. This area of the tooth is usually under the gum tissue in patients that have had minimal bone loss in the area.

77. B: Dental hand piece fiber optics should only be cleaned with a minimally abrasive cleaning solution, such as isopropyl alcohol. Cleaning the fiber optics with lubricating oil is not recommended as the lubricating oil is to be used on the ports on the hand piece, as directed by the manufacturer. A wire brush should never be used when cleaning a hand piece of any kind, as the wire bristles will scratch the delicate fiber optics of the hand piece.

78. C: In order for private health information regarding a specific patient to be released, the recipient must be a family member who is directly responsible for providing care to the patient, another healthcare provider or specialist involved in providing care to the patient, or an attorney or law enforcement official required by the state or a court order. Otherwise, private healthcare information may not be released without the patient's approval.

79. B: Fluoride is a mineral that helps keep teeth healthy by preventing tooth decay. Some water supplies are fluoridated; however, patients who do not have fluoridated water will require some form of fluoride supplements. Professionally applied fluoride is often indicated for some children. Fluoride gels or foam are commonly used for this purpose. The fluoride is placed in the disposable tray. The patient must be seated in an upright position to help prevent fluoride from accidently being swallowed. The teeth are dried using the air-water syringe. The tray is put into the mouth and the patient is instructed to bite down. The fluoride is squeezed over the teeth. The saliva ejector is used to clean out the saliva so the fluoride is not swallowed. After the appropriate application time, the saliva ejector is used to remove the saliva and fluoride. The patient should not rinse the mouth or eat or drink anything for at least 30 minutes in order to maximize the effectiveness of the fluoride treatment.

80. B: Periotomes are instruments used for severing the periodontal ligament during periodontal surgery. They are most commonly used during extractions of the tooth or root. The periotome should be inserted into the periodontal space to sever the periodontal ligament and then gently moved around the root to extract the root and tooth from the space.

81. C: Boxing wax is the type of wax that is placed around the outer edges or periphery of an impression and allows for a wall to be formed. This wall will then be used to hold in the gypsum product used to pour up the impression to produce the end model of the teeth. Baseplate wax is used during denture construction to hold artificial teeth in place, inlay wax is used to make patterns on a die of a tooth, and casting wax is used to make wax patterns for partial denture frameworks.

82. A: There are many different types of dental insurance. Each type may use a different method for calculating fees for service benefits, including fixed fee schedule, schedule of benefits, and UCR (usual, customary, and reasonable) fees. A deductible is the amount of money that must be paid towards the insurer's dental treatment before the insurance benefits will be activated. A copayment is the way dental treatment fees are split between the insurance carrier and the insured. Many carriers will split 80/20, where the insurance covers 80% and the insured must pay 20% of the total fee. Benefit eligibility is the term used to determine if the insured is able to start receiving benefits. New employees typically have to wait 30 to 60 days before benefits are activated. Many insurance carriers will require a pretreatment estimate or predetermination of benefits before any substantial dental work is initiated to make sure the patient and dentist are aware of the coverage that is available.

83. C: During application of dental sealants, the dental assistant must carefully dispense the sealant material and gently work the material into the grooves and fissures. If the material is applied too quickly, or if there is excessive manipulation and scrubbing of the sealant when on the tooth, air bubbles can form causing holes to appear in the surface of the sealant.

84. C: Removing bone from one area of the body and moving it to another is known as bone grafting. There are different types of bone grafts, depending on where the donor tissue originates. Tissue taken from the patient's own mouth and grafted to a different location is known as autologous graft. Tissue taken from a donor, either someone known to the patient or an anonymous donor is an allogenic graft.

85. C: "T-Bands" are primarily used during restorative procedures that include the restoration of deciduous teeth. Tofflemire matrix bands are used primarily during the restoration on interproximal surfaces on adult teeth. During a pulpectomy procedure, the objective is to remove a portion of the pulp that is abnormal or has become invaded by decay. Prophylactic appointments for both adult and children allow the dentist or hygienist to clean the teeth and remove excess debris to facilitate good oral hygiene.

86. D: When preparing to mix calcium hydroxide as a liner, a small amount of both the base and catalyst should be expressed on a small mixing pad. If both the base and the catalyst aren't placed onto the mixing pad, the reaction will not occur. Dental tray adhesives are not used in conjunction with calcium hydroxide. Dental adhesives are primarily used to provide added adhesion within a dental impression tray to hold the impression material in place. Because such a small quantity of the calcium hydroxide will be needed as a liner, using a large mixing pad is wasteful to the dental practice.

87. D: A dental office needs to take precautions to ensure that the patient information it is dealing with is kept private. This includes not placing patient schedules up around the office, keeping patient charts locked up when not in use, and not allowing patients to have views or access to other patients' charts or information, as well as placing copy and fax machines in areas where the information being copied or faxed is not visible to others.

88. D: Expendable supplies are supplies including cotton rolls, restorative materials, and impression materials that are commonly used in a dental office and are replaced often. Due to the frequent use of these supplies, they must always be available for dental team members to use, so having a good inventory management system is crucial in a dental office.

89. C: The surgical curette is the instrument used following an extraction to rid the extraction site of any diseased tissue or abscessed areas. This instrument comes in a variety of sizes to allow for the working end to be able to fit into a wide range of extraction sites.

90. B: When taking a patient's blood pressure, ensure the patient is seated with legs and arms uncrossed. The dental assistant should place the cuff slightly above the elbow, inflate the cuff slowly, and once it reaches capacity, allow the air to slowly escape the cuff while listening to blood flow through the brachial artery.

91. B: A class III restoration is one that involves the interproximal surface of the anterior teeth. Composite material would be the material of choice when performing this type of restoration because it is malleable and the correct color choice can be selected. A crown is not needed for a class III restoration, and amalgam material would produce discoloration of the tooth.

92. A: The malposition of a tooth that tips toward the direction of the cheek is known as buccoversion. A tooth that is not in alignment with the adjacent teeth in its quadrant, but rather tips toward the lingual is said to be in linguoversion.

93. D: The plastic instrument is used during a composite restoration to allow the dentist to place the composite material into a prepared tooth and is not used during an amalgam procedure. During an amalgam procedure, the dental assistant will load an amalgam carrier with amalgam and transfer this to the dentist, followed by the condenser.

94. C: When dental assistants are working under general supervision, they are able to perform specific tasks that have been authorized by the dentist without the dentist having to be physically present at the dental clinic. This is different from other levels of supervision because the dentist does not need to be at the office, although in the other levels the dentist does need to be physically present.

95. A: Older patients have a higher prevalence of root surface decay due to the recession of gum tissue and bone that commonly occurs with aging. The root surface of a tooth is not covered by enamel and therefore is not protected like the coronal surface of a tooth is, leaving this area more susceptible to decay.

Share Your Story!

It's Your Moment, Let's Celebrate It!

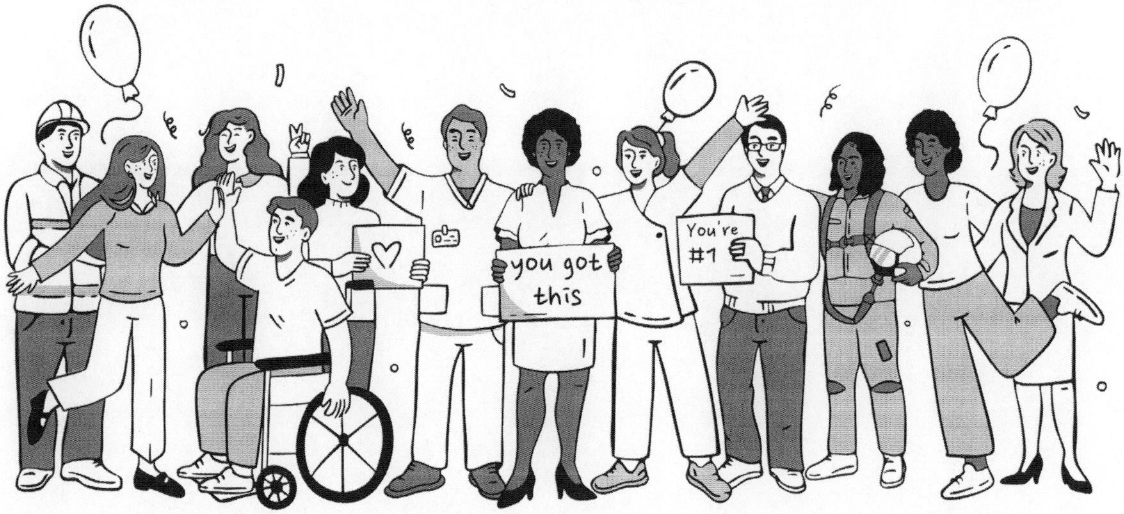

Share your story @mometrixtestpreparation